Psychiatry for nurses

Psychiatry for nurses

JOHN GIBSON
MD FRCPsych DPM

FOURTH EDITION

BLACKWELL SCIENTIFIC PUBLICATIONS
OXFORD LONDON EDINBURGH MELBOURNE

© 1962, 1965, 1971, 1979 by
Blackwell Scientific Publications
Editorial Offices:
Osney Mead, Oxford, OX2 0EL
8 John Street, London, WC1N 2ES
9 Forrest Road, Edinburgh,
   EH1 2QH
214 Berkeley Street, Carlton
   Victoria 3053, Australia

First published 1962
Second edition 1965
Third edition 1971
Fourth edition 1979

Phototypeset in V.I.P. Plantin by
Western Printing Services Ltd,
Bristol
Printed and bound in Great Britain
by
Billing & Sons Ltd,
Guildford, London and Worcester

DISTRIBUTORS
USA
   Blackwell Mosby Book
   Distributors
   11830 Westline Industrial Drive
   St Louis, Missouri 63141

Canada
   Blackwell Mosby Book
   Distributors
   86 Northline Road, Toronto
   Ontario, M4B 3E5

Australia
   Blackwell Scientific Book
   Distributors
   214 Berkeley Street, Carlton
   Victoria 3053

British Library
Cataloguing in Publication Data

Gibson, John, b. 1907
   Psychiatry for nurses. - 4th ed.
   1. Psychiatry
   2. Psychiatric nursing
   I. Title
   616.8'9'0024613   RC454

ISBN 0-632-00597-1

Contents

Preface to fourth edition

For this edition the book has been thoroughly revised and extensively rewritten in order to bring it up to date and to present much of the material in tabular form for easy learning.

Chapter 1 · The scope of psychiatry

Psychiatry is the branch of medicine that concerns itself with mental illness and mental handicap. It tries to understand the causes of these conditions, to describe them, to discover their frequency, to prevent them, and to cure or improve people suffering from them.

There is no clear distinction between mental illness and physical illness. What distinction there is has largely arisen because a mental illness is liable to produce such an abnormality of the patient's behaviour that it is difficult to treat him at home or in a ward in a general hospital. Patients with mental illnesses came to be treated in mental hospitals, and doctors and nurses who look after patients with physical illnesses did not have much to do with them. The situation has now changed. General hospitals have wards and outpatient departments for psychiatric patients. The change coincided with the introduction of some modern methods of treatment which shortened some mental illnesses and so improved the behaviour of many patients that it became possible to look after them under conditions of greater freedom.

The general nurse in the course of her general nursing will already have met some mental abnormalities. During a fever a patient can become confused, express absurd ideas or act strangely. A young febrile child can have a fit. A patient with a cerebral tumour can become dull, absent-minded and forgetful. With myxoedema a patient is dull, apathetic and indifferent to his surroundings. With thyrotoxicosis a patient is nervous, anxious and tense. Many a patient with a physical illness becomes worried, depressed and even suicidal, and sometimes a patient with a serious disease, such as multiple sclerosis or pulmonary tuberculosis, is morbidly happy, imagining that he is not ill or is getting better. As she gains experience of psychiatric conditions the nurse will learn that mentally ill patients are not essentially different from physically ill patients, that they suffer from illnesses of known type, with a definite course like any physical illness, that definite methods of treatment are applicable to many of them.

Psychiatric disorders are usually classified under three main headings:

psychoses,
neuroses,
mental handicap.

The divisions between these types are not exact ones.

Psychoses

The psychoses are the insanities—the sorts of illness for which a patient was likely to be admitted into a mental hospital. The most common are schizophrenia, affective states, dementia, and those mental illnesses known to be produced by disease or injury of the brain. Many patients with this kind of illness are severely disturbed in their thoughts or behaviour.

Neuroses

Neuroses are usually milder illnesses than the psychoses and do not produce such severe disturbance of thought and behaviour. The common neuroses are anxiety state, hysteria, and obsessional-compulsive state.

Mental handicap

Mental handicap (retardation) is the condition in which the person is so much below average intelligence that he requires special education, training or control. There are varying degrees of mental handicap, from at the lowest level a helpless person who is unable to look after himself in any way to the person who only just fails to cope with the demands for work and behaviour that society places upon him.

In addition to these main groups are several conditions that cannot easily be classified.

Psychopathy is not easy to define and different doctors include different conditions under the heading. It is used to describe both those who are abnormally aggressive or seriously irresponsible and also drug addicts, alcoholics, eccentric and sexually abnormal people.

Psychosomatic disorders are conditions in which emotional factors are thought to play a large part in their production or continuation, e.g. asthma, peptic ulcer, ulcerative colitis.

Epilepsy can be considered as both a psychiatric and a neurological problem.

The *psychiatry of childhood* is concerned with the special psychiatric problems presented by children, e.g. autism, stammering, bed-wetting.

A patient can suffer from more than one psychiatric condition. Symptoms characteristic of a neurosis may hide a psychosis, which in time emerges and is recognizable. An alcoholic man may be alcoholic because he is primarily a depressive, a manic or an epileptic. A mentally handicapped person can develop a neurosis or a psychosis.

The *causes* of psychiatric illnesses are numerous and complex. They include genetic abnormalities, degenerations of brain cells, infections by viruses and other organisms, interference with the cerebral blood supply, emotional stress, deprivation of love, and faulty upbringing in childhood.

The recognition that a person is mentally ill can be easy or difficult. It is easy when he expresses very abnormal ideas or is very disturbed in behaviour. It is difficult when symptoms are not obvious, as at the beginning of a slowly developing illness. It is important to know something of the previous personality of the patient. Was he happy or discontented? Was he careful or careless? Was he intelligent or dull? Was he stable or unstable? Was he a loner or a mixer? A slight difference in personality is often the first indication of the onset of a mental illness. The patient himself may lack insight—he may not appreciate that he is in any way abnormal, and insisting that he is quite well refuse to accept treatment or advice.

A *psychiatrist* is a doctor who practises psychiatry.

A *psychotherapist* is a person who treats patients by psychotherapy, by psychological methods and not by physical methods. He is usually a doctor, but not necessarily one. He may be a psychologist. He is more likely to treat neurotics and children than psychotics.

A *psychoanalyst* is a psychotherapist engaged in the practice of psychoanalysis. The two principal kinds are Freudian analysts, who work on the principles laid down by Sigmund Freud

(1856–1939), an Austrian doctor, and Jungian analysts, who work on the principles laid down by Carl G. Jung (1875–1961), a Swiss doctor. A *lay analyst* is one who is not medically qualified.

A *psychologist* is a person trained in the study of mental processes and behaviour. Usually he is not medically qualified and has a university degree in psychology and has specialized in clinical, educational or industrial psychology.

A new and exciting development for nurses was initiated in 1972 when a small group of psychiatric nurses began training to become *nurse therapists*. This highly specialized training is now available at three centres in the United Kingdom. Nurse therapists use behavioural therapy and other dynamic psychotherapeutic techniques to treat a wide range of adult neurotic disorders.

Chapter 2 · Symptoms and signs of mental disease

Mental illness can begin slowly or suddenly. When it begins suddenly symptoms are usually severe and it is obvious that the patient is ill. But if an illness begins slowly, arising out of the patient's personality, it may be impossible to say when it began. The study of a person's personality is important in two ways: (a) it is an indication of the sort of illness he is likely to develop, and (b) a slight change in his personality may be the first sign that something is wrong with him. The taking of a history is important for it is often possible to make the diagnosis from the history alone. In the assessment of a patient it is important to learn as much as possible of his personality and background, of his place in society and of the standards of his society. What might be permissible for a navvy might suggest mental illness in a bishop; what a small boy did might be suspect if a middle-aged man did it.

General conduct

If a person develops a mental illness, his conduct is likely to deviate from his norm. A friendly man could become aloof, cold and suspicious. The quiet solitary man could become hearty. A man might develop a deep interest in unusual religions or societies. He might give up his work, interests and hobbies. A patient with a severe mental illness can neglect his personal hygiene and clothing. In acute mental illness a patient can tear his clothes and expose himself. In chronic mental illness a patient tends to cling to the style of dress fashionable at the time he broke down, or dresses himself in unusual ways and decorates himself with badges, brooches and trifles.

Eating

In many mental illnesses patients eat less. A patient may not eat because he is too excited, because he is deluded that food is

5

poisoned, because he is depressed and wishes to die, because he has an obsession to slim. Worried people can eat too much and become fat. Alcohol may be drunk to excess by excited patients, depressed patients, or by patients with early organic disease of the brain.

Sleep

Insomnia is common in mental illness. A patient may have difficulty in getting to sleep, he may wake early, he may have nightmares. A very excited patient may get no natural sleep. Old people may show 'inverted sleep rhythm'—sleeping by day and being awake at night.

Activity

In a state of excitement a patient is likely to do more than he usually does and to do it carelessly and with little regard for other people; he may begin one thing before he has finished another and leave behind him a trail of unfinished projects. Another patient may do less than he normally does because of loss of interest, of a feeling that the job is not worth doing, or of lack of appreciation that the work is to be done. An obsessional patient is compelled to repeat a task from a fear that he has not done it satisfactorily.

Stereotypy is the repetition of an act, as a depressed patient may wring his hands or go on beating himself.

Perseveration is the repetition of words spoken or actions performed in spite of the patient's efforts to do or say something else.

Negativism is the doing of the opposite the patient is told to do, or is used to describe the behaviour of a patient who does what he should not, e.g. spitting out food, refusing to wash, retaining urine and faeces.

Automatic obedience is the automatic obedience of an order, whether it is sensible or not.

Echolalia is the repetition of anything that is said: if the nurse says, 'How are you today?', the patient replies with 'How are you today?'

Echopraxia is the repetition by the patient of any action that is performed in front of him: if the nurse crosses her hands, the patient crosses his.

Flexibilitas cerea (waxy flexibility) is the willingness of the patient to allow himself or his limbs to be placed in any position and keep them there.

Emotional changes

Normal people show normal changes of mood—becoming happy when things are going well for them and unhappy when they are going badly. Some rigid personalities do not show much mood change. Others have a cyclothymic personality, with a swing of mood between happiness and sadness.

Euphoria is a feeling of well-being.

Elation is a feeling of great well-being and happiness.

Depression is a feeling of sadness, varying from mild to severe, and in its most severe form *depressive stupor* develops.

Incongruity of affect is an inappropriate mood, e.g. giggling or laughing in a serious condition.

Disturbances of thought

Disturbances of thought consist of too few thoughts, too many thoughts, or abnormal thoughts.

Poverty of ideas is a reduction of thought below that of the person's normal state: he can think of little or nothing, or thoughts are blocked from coming fully into consciousness.

Flight of ideas is the state in which one thought after another rushes through the patient's mind, thoughts which seem not to be connected, but which have a connection in the patient's mind. There may be a *clang association*—an association of ideas by the sound and not by the sense.

Ideas of reference are ideas the patient has that people are referring to him by their remarks or gestures, by references in the media, etc.

Delusions are false beliefs. Delusions are commonly of persecution: the patient believes that people are talking about him, following him, spying on him, poisoning his food, turning rays of all kinds on him, trying to kill him or drive him insane. *Nihilistic delusions* are delusions that one no longer exists, either completely or in part, that one is dead or has never been alive. *Delusions of grandeur* are less common than delusions of persecution. They take the form of believing that one is more powerful, mighty, wealthy or beautiful than one is. The patient may believe that he is a millionaire, the strongest man in the world, a king, a TV star.

Hallucinations are sensory impressions without external stimuli to cause them. The commonest hallucinations are auditory: the patient hears sounds or voices. Sounds may be clear or vague, ringing or buzzing or of music. Hallucinatory voices are usually abusive, threatening and accusatory, and sound very real to the patient, who feels himself committed to obeying them. Sometimes he identifies the voices as coming from a particular person, whom he may attack or complain of to the police.

Visual hallucinations are of shapes, faces or people. Lilliputian hallucinations are hallucinations of tiny people. Hallucinations of smell, taste and touch are less common. Hallucinations of smell and taste may cause a person to believe that he is being drugged or poisoned.

Hypnogogic hallucinations are hallucinations occurring in the drowsy state between walking and sleeping; they are like dreams and a person may on awakening realize what they are.

Ideas of depersonalization are ideas that a person's body is being altered in some way, that one is not quite real or cannot feel real sensations or emotions. *Ideas of derealization* are that the world has become strange, unreal, unnatural.

Disturbances of speech

In *flight of ideas* one idea is expressed very quickly after another without the listener being able to follow them or to see any connection between them. *Circumstantiality* is talking in great detail about a subject and wandering round it without actually leaving it. *Neologisms* are new words invented by the speaker. *Word-salad* is a meaningless jumble of words.

Blocking of the stream of talk is a stoppage of talk which the speaker cannot explain or prevent. In *mutism* the speaker does not talk at all, although physically capable of doing so.

Disturbances of consciousness

A patient with a mental illness may be fully conscious of all that is going on around him, or he may have some degree of impairment of consciousness.

Disorientation is a faulty appreciation of time, place or person. If he is disorientated in time, he does not know what hour of the day it is, what day of the week it is, and so on; if he is disorientated in place he does not know where he is; if he is disorientated in person he does not know who he is.

In *confusion* the patient is imperfectly aware of what is going on, is muddled in his thoughts and possibly deluded and hallucinated. In *delirium* he is acutely confused with contact with reality lost or almost completely lost. *Stupor* is the condition in which the patient lies apparently oblivious of what is going on around him, and not eating, drinking or excreting; although apparently oblivious, he may be aware of what is going on around him, may be misinterpreting it and living in a life of phantasy, and on arousing from stupor he may be able to recall in detail what has been said to him or done in front of him. In *coma* the patient is unconscious and cannot be aroused by stimuli.

Disturbances of intelligence

A person's intelligence increases in early life, but after the age of about eighteen there is no further increase in 'pure' intelligence. One's intelligence varies with the amount of intellectual pressure put upon one, and a child brought up by dull parents can appear duller than he is because he lacks stimulation. In later years people show a varying decline in intelligence. Some show little change, others a definite decline, with loss of memory, inability to cope with new problems, and difficulty in adjusting to new situations.

Amnesia is loss of memory. It can be for recent events, for distant events, or 'global' i.e. for everything. *Confabulation* is the invention of events and remarks to fill up gaps in memory.

Folie à deux is the occurrence of the same mental symptoms in two people living closely together, e.g. husband and wife, mother and daughter, sister and sister. Folie à trois (three) and greater numbers can occur.

Criminal or antisocial behaviour

Criminal or antisocial behaviour is often produced by mental illness or handicap, and this can make the assessment of responsibility very difficult. Mentally handicapped people may not have sufficient intelligence to appreciate what they are doing and the consequences of their actions. Deluded or hallucinated people can assault or kill people they imagine are persecuting or abusing them. Depressed people can commit or attempt suicide or murder their families. Organic deterioration of the brain can lead people to expose themselves, get drunk, commit sexual crimes, drive cars recklessly, or cause fires. Alcoholism is a common cause of driving and swimming accidents. Drug addiction can cause abnormal behaviour.

Chapter 3 · The neuroses

The neuroses are:

>anxiety states,
>hysteria,
>obsessive-compulsive states.

They are conditions characterized by disturbances of thought processes, of emotional reactions, of behaviour, and of—in many patients—physical functions.

The neuroses are contrasted with the psychoses. The distinction is often difficult to make, and patients with a psychosis can show symptoms characteristic of a neurosis. In general, the neurotic patient remains in touch with his environment, while the psychotic becomes more and more out of touch with it. A severe neurosis can, however, be as disabling as a psychosis.

Anxiety states

An anxiety state is a condition in which a patient shows excessive anxiety, often associated with evidence of overactivity of the autonomic nervous system.

I. PREDISPOSING FACTORS.

Anxiety to some degree is a normal reaction. Everyone develops anxiety when faced with great difficulties and danger. In a normal person these reactions are natural, and everyone has a breaking point at which he breaks down. In an anxiety state the patient's reactions are excessive, prolonged beyond the time of the emergency, or without obvious cause.

The patient with an anxiety state is likely to have been brought up in an atmosphere of anxiety at home. One or both of his parents may have responded with anxiety to any domestic difficulty, have worried about the health or progress of their children or have overprotected them and restricted their activities needlessly. In consequence, the child learns that anxiety is the response to trouble. Healthy children are likely to have fears—of the dark, of being alone, of animals, of thunder and lightning. The anxious child shows these fears to excess and has other fears, and does not grow out of them like the healthy child.

A patient may attribute his first attack to a specific event. This can be an operation or accident, and less commonly a separation, a fright, the birth of a sibling, loss of income or job.

2. ACUTE ANXIETY STATE

An acute anxiety state is precipitated by a sudden, severe stress. The patient is likely to show:

increased heart rate,	precordial discomfort or pain,
rapid respiratory rate,	hyperventilation,
diarrhoea,	urgency of micturition,
choking feeling,	dilated pupils,
sweating,	tremor of hands.
dry mouth,	

His face expresses his anxiety, he may feel totally exhausted, and he may become completely immobilized. He may be unable to sleep, and what sleep he gets is likely to be disturbed by nightmares.

An acute anxiety state can last from minutes to days. In a person of good personality who has broken down under intolerable stress complete recovery is likely.

3. CHRONIC ANXIETY STATE

A chronic anxiety state can be chronic from the beginning or can follow an acute anxiety state. In it the patient is chronically worried, with the severity of his symptoms varying without completely clearing up. He may worry about anything, many of his worries being centred in the physical manifestations of the associated autonomic overactivity. Anxiety is said to be 'fixated' when it is focused on a particular part of the body, such as the head, stomach or chest, of whose allegedly irregular functioning the patient complains intensely.

The patient is likely to complain of some of the following:

palpitations,	giddiness,
blackouts,	sweating,

diarrhoea,	fullness in the stomach,
fatigue,	urgency and frequency of
sleeping badly,	micturition,
irregular heart action,	fear of going insane,
fainting,	stammering.
tremors,	

His anxiety can be attached to a specific situation. In *claustrophobia* he is afraid of closed spaces and may be unable to go into a bus or cinema. In *agoraphobia* he is afraid of open spaces and may be unable to walk alone across a square or through a field; one form of this is the *housebound syndrome*, in which the patient, usually a woman, has not been out of doors for years.

An *effort syndrome* is an anxiety state with emphasis on the circulatory system, the patient complaining of palpitations, precordial pain, pounding of the heart, irregularity of the heart, and shortness of breath. It occurs in persons of asthenic build with a small heart and an inadequate personality when they have to engage in hard physical work under stress.

4. TREATMENT

(a) *Acute anxiety state*. The patient should be removed from the stress-producing situation and given sedation, sometimes for several days. Abreation techniques may be used. (b) *Chronic anxiety state*. Treatment is unsatisfactory. The patient's personality is not likely to be changeable; and as his condition is likely to get better or worse spontaneously, it is difficult to assess the value of any particular treatment. Psychotherapy by simple reassurance and suggestion may be helpful. An attempt may be made to 'desensitize' the patient from the stress-producing situation. Tranquillizers are given to allay anxiety and agitation. Modified insulin treatment is given for severe cases.

Hysteria

Hysteria appears in many forms and can stimulate the signs and symptoms of physical diseases. In it psychological stresses produce disturbances of function or disturbances of behaviour and consciousness.

1. HYSTERICAL PERSONALITY

Hysteria is most likely to occur in a person with a hysterical personality. The patient is usually a woman. The person with this personality is immature, dependent upon others, over-reacting and given to self-display. With a persistence of infantile trends and an immature psychosexual development, she may live in childish daydreams.

There is often a family history of hysterical reaction, unreliability and unstable behaviour.

2. PRECIPITATING FACTORS

A hysterical illness may be precipitated by stress, an accident or a physical illness. It may occur when a person is exposed to a stimulus to which he could react in two ways, e.g. a soldier in great danger might be divided between fighting and running away (the 'fight or flight' syndrome). Hysterical features can also occur in other illnesses—in epilepsy, schizophrenia, depression, anxiety state, and any organic disease of the brain.

3. CLINICAL FEATURES

A patient usually shows several features of the illness, either at the same time or at different times. Clinical features fall generally into two main groups:

(a) *conversion reactions*: there is a disturbance of physical function,
(b) *dissociative reactions*: there is a disturbance of consciousness memory and behaviour.

The patient may display *la belle indifférence*—a lack of concern for her disability, e.g. regarding a paralysed limb as if it were a matter of no importance. She leaves the fussing and worrying to be done by her relatives. She may have outbursts of tantrums.

4. CONVERSION REACTIONS

Paralysis. A flaccid or spastic paralysis can occur. Usually one limb or part of one limb is affected. The tendon reflexes and electrical reactions of muscle are normal, and there is no atrophy unless paralysis has been present for a long time. A spastic paralysis can produce contractures.

The patient may have a peculiar gait, unlike that produced by a physical disease. A flaccid leg is dragged or a spastic leg is flung with irregular movements in all directions.

Hysterical aphonia. The patient is unable to speak except in a whisper.

Hysterical mutism. The patient is unable to make any sound, but she may be able to express herself in writing or gestures.

Hysterical stammering. The patient stammers and has spasms of the lips, tongue and pharynx.

Anaesthesia. Usually this is a diminution of sensation in a limb or part of a limb. Both superficial and deep sensation can be lost. The anaesthesia may be limited to the area covered by a glove, sock or stocking, and is not related to the distribution of sensory nerves, which does not accord with this pattern. If the body is involved, anaesthesia can stop dead at the midline, there being none of the slight overlap of sensation over the midline. The mucous membrane of mouth, throat, rectum and vagina may become anaesthetic.

Pains and paraesthesiae. Painful and tender spots can be present, or the patient may complain of itching, burning, and indescribable sensations.

Hyperaesthesia of the scalp can cause headache. Recurrent abdominal pain may have caused the patient to undergo surgical operations.

Hysterical blindness and deafness. Hysterical blindness can come on and disappear suddenly, and is associated with blepharospasm and photophobia. There can be complete blindness or constriction of the fields of vision as if the patient were looking down a tube. On physical examination the eyes appear normal, and the patient does not walk into danger or bump into people. Hysterical deafness of long or short duration can occur.

Visceral manifestations. These include attacks of rapid breathing or rapid heart action, blushing and blanching of the skin, diarrhoea, vomiting, belching, the production of abdominal noises, the expulsion of large amounts of flatus, constipation, and raising the temperature by several degrees.

5. DISSOCIATIVE REACTIONS

These reactions are liable to occur in the hysterical, unstable, early schizophrenia and psychopathy. They are liable to occur when the patient is in serious trouble, and the diagnosis from malingering is difficult.

Hysterical amnesia. This can be complete or incomplete, or limited to certain events and people in the patient's life. The patient may be unable to recognize his relatives and may deny that he has seen them before.

Fugue. This is a 'twilight' state in which the patient wanders about with a partially clouded consciousness, neglecting himself, sometimes without eating, and turning up somewhere without being able to give any account of himself.

Hysterical trance. The patient lies in a state outwardly resembling sleep, with anaesthesia for ordinary stimuli. The attack ends with the patient having an amnesia for it.

Somnambulism (sleep-walking). Without waking up the patient gets out of bed and wanders about. He may stay in the house or go out into the street, or start to do some work. He may put himself back to bed or wake up where he is.

Normal children may occasionally sleep-walk.

Ganser syndrome. This is sometimes seen in prisoners, in schizophrenics and in patients with cerebral tumour. It is called the 'syndrome of approximate answers'. The patient goes into a dull, stupid state, and when asked questions gives answers that are off the point.

Munchausen syndrome. This term is used to describe persons who get themselves admitted to hospital over and over again, giving a history of an acute medical or surgical crisis, submit to investigation or operation, and discharge themselves. The patient may have shown gross hysterical manifestation, or been in mental hospital or prison.

6. TREATMENT

The treatment of hysteria is very difficult. The patient has a personality that is unlikely to change, and symptoms appear and disappear inexplicably.

An acute hysterical state is likely to respond to removal from a stress-producing situation, rest, sedation and supportive psychotherapy. Hypnosis may be useful in removing a particular feature such as aphonia or a paralysis; but as the basic personality is unaffected, the disappearance of one symptom is likely to be followed by the appearance of another. Behavioural therapy is likely to be helpful only when the patient and therapist agree to work on one particular problem at a time and when the problem and aim of the treatment are agreed.

Obsessional-compulsive neurosis

In this neurosis the patient is compelled to think or behave repetitively and cannot stop himself from doing so.

Obsessional-compulsive features can occur in children, and many children go through periods when they have to think certain thoughts or behave in certain ways. Some adults have compulsions such as turning back to see if the gas taps are turned off. The patient with this neurosis is likely to be the child of obsessional parents and to have been brought up to be very clean and tidy and toilet-trained at too early an age. In consequence he is well behaved usually, but he can have temper tantrums in which he wants to kill the parent who has made him conform.

The neurosis develops in adult life. Usually no precipitating factor is found. There is a wide range of obsessional ideas and compulsive actions. Obsessional thoughts of being dirty are common, driving the patient to compulsive washing. Some patients are obsessed with the thought that they are going to utter blasphemous or obscene words. Others may be obsessed with numbers or with their personal appearance. Books and papers may have to be kept in particular order and not moved. Furniture or fences may have to be touched as they are passed. Occasionally a patient will pass through an acute depressive episode.

The obsessional thoughts and compulsive actions may be symbolic representations of desires the patient cannot consciously accept, or they may be punishments for thoughts and actions about which he has unconscious guilt. They are often accompanied by anxiety and guilt feelings. Obsessional ideas also occur in depression and early schizophrenia. Occasionally a chronic obsessional patient develops schizophrenia.

TREATMENT

Assessment of treatment is difficult for a patient's symptoms can get better or worse without obvious cause. Spontaneous remissions can occur. Supportive psychotherapy is given. Tranquillizers, such as chlorpromazine (Largactil) are given to relieve anxiety. Leucotomy may be used for a severe chronic obsessional-compulsive, whose condition has not been relieved by other treatment.

Chapter 4 · Psychosomatic diseases

The psychosomatic diseases are those 'physical' diseases of which psychological factors are thought to be predominating and perpetuating factors.

Emotional factors are known to produce minor symptoms such as:

vague pains,	headache,
palpitations,	dyspepsia,
diarrhoea,	frequency of micturition,
sweating,	rapid heart rate,
blushing,	blanching.

It is argued that emotional factors can produce longer-lasting disturbances and chronic physical changes in tissues. Among the diseases in which psychosomatic factors are thought to be components are:

anorexia nervosa,	peptic ulcer,
ulcerative colitis,	asthma,
hypertension,	coronary thrombosis,
multiple sclerosis,	hyperthyroidism.
eczema and other skin diseases,	

Any chronic, unpleasant, painful and repetitive disease is, however, likely to produce psychological effects on the patient which are a reaction to his illness and not a cause of it.

The factors in any psychosomatic disease are as follows.

1. It is produced and made worse by emotion.
2. It is liable to disappear and return.
3. The patient has a particular type of personality.
4. The patient may suffer from more than one psychosomatic disease at the same time or at different times.
5. There is likely to be a family history of such diseases.

Anorexia nervosa

This is a disease mainly of adolescent girls and young women. It occurs much less commonly in children, older women and men.

Cause. No definite cause is known.

Personality and psychological factors. The patient may have shown neurotic traits in earlier life. She may have a poorly integrated personality, or have been over-conscientious. She is likely to be of average or above average intelligence and to come from the upper social classes. She may have had spells of overeating or been liable to rapid fluctuations in weight.

She is likely to be attached to her father and resentful of her mother. The mother may be fat and the patient does not wish to be like her; she may have an unconscious fear of pregnancy, or she may associate obesity with sexuality.

CLINICAL FEATURES

The patient gives up eating in adequate amounts, and in consequence becomes slim and even emaciated. She develops a great aversion for food, she may feel sick at the mention or sight of it, and she may vomit if she is forced to eat. She may have food fads, always preferring those of little nutritional value.

In addition to the severe loss of weight she is likely to show:

    amenorrhoea,
    anaemia,
    constipation,
    a downy growth of hair on
        the skin.

The patient can be bright and active and go for long, fast, solitary walks. She may strongly express her reasons for not eating. On the other hand, she may be irritable, depressed and have various phobias and obsessions, and she may have abnormal ideas about her body-image, insisting that she is too fat. Some patients become shop-lifters of unsuitable food.

The disease varies in severity and length. Some women recover completely with weight about normal, regular menstruation, reasonably good mental state, and a satisfactory social, sexual and work record. Some do not recover completely and are left with some degree of 'weight phobia', irregular or absent menstruation, depression, and inadequate social and sexual adjustment. A few go on to dangerous emaciation and die of starvation or secondary infection.

Factors which suggest that the prognosis is poor or bad are:

a long illness,
very low weight,
poor parental relationships,
poor adjustment in childhood,
older age of onset,
vomiting.

TREATMENT

The patient has usually to be admitted into hospital because the necessary control cannot be maintained at home, the family's patience having been worn out or the mother converted to the daughter's views on food.

The patient should be nursed in bed until her weight is back to normal. Strict nursing care is essential. Every attempt should be made to persuade the patient to eat normally. If she gets the opportunity she will hide food, put it out of the window or flush it down the lavatory. One of the nurse's jobs is to see that the patient actually eats the food she is given and does not dispose of it in some other way.

The food should be of good nutritional value and additional vitamin supplements should be given.

The patient should be weighed nude twice a week. If she is weighed in her clothes, she will try to hide in them something heavy to give the impression that she is gaining weight. Tube feeding can sometimes be necessary.

The doctor may try some kind of psychotherapy.

Drug treatment by tranquillizers is often used.

Other kinds of treatment used include ECT and leucotomy.

Peptic ulcer

A peptic ulcer is a localized ulceration of the gastric or duodenal wall directly produced by the digestion of the wall by gastric juice, and liable to heal, recur and become chronic. Why the mucous membrane and sometimes the rest of the stomach or duodenal wall should be digested in this way is unknown.

The type of person who develops a peptic ulcer and possible precipitating factors have been studied. An ulcer is said to occur predominantly in a person whose ambition, hard work, aggression and rigidity hide a personality that is basically infantile, with strong infantile demands for care and protection. The precipitating factor may be prolonged frustration and anxiety, and further stress can cause an ulcer to reappear or become worse. Tranquillizers, simple psychotherapy, and if possible improvements in the environment are used in treatment.

Ulcerative colitis

Ulcerative colitis is an inflammatory disease of the colon, which can occur at any age, but most commonly begins in early adult life; there may be a family history. Recurrent attacks of inflammation produce bleeding from the bowel, diarrhoea, abdominal pain, emaciation and fever. The disease can run an acute or chronic course, with improvement, exacerbations and recurrences; it can cause death.

It is said to occur particularly in people who are emotionally unstable, obsessional or introverted. It has been precipitated or made worse by an unexpected bereavement, loss of job, or separation from a loved or controlling person. Tranquillizers and psychotherapy have a part to play in treatment.

Asthma

Asthma is characterized by attacks of wheezing and difficult breathing, due to a spasm of the muscle in the bronchi. In many cases an attack is precipitated by an allergic factor, and the patient may show other allergic conditions such as hay fever and eczema.

Psychological factors are important in the precipitation of attacks. In childhood attacks are precipitated by emotional stresses, such as parental overprotection, rejection, anxiety in parents who strive for perfection in their children. In later life attacks are precipitated by stress and anxiety, by threats to security, by bereavement, sexual and marital problems, financial difficulties, assaults and frights. Fear of an attack is an added and justified complication.

Relieving emotional stresses, improving parental attitudes and making environmental improvements are factors in the prevention of attacks.

Hypertension

Hypertension is a disease for which often no cause can be found; some types are secondary to kidney disease, narrowing of the aorta, narrowing of renal arteries, etc.

The affected person is said to have a personality that is outwardly ambitious, energetic and ruthless, and inwardly seething with resentment and hostility. The raised blood pressure is thus the product of emotional stress in a person of strong drives and equally strong frustration. Doubt has been expressed, however, whether persons with hypertension show a particular personality pattern.

Coronary thrombosis

Coronary thrombosis is a clotting of blood in the coronary arteries, which supply the heart with blood.

The personality of the person who is liable to develop a coronary thrombosis is said to be one of over-carefulness about work and time, an insistence on over-work, an inability to relax and feelings of guilt when not working. An attack can be precipitated by the association of unaccustomed hard work with an anxiety-producing situation.

Multiple sclerosis

Multiple (disseminated) sclerosis is a disease of the central nervous system in which there are recurrent attacks of acute inflammation in patches; with healing, areas affected can become fibrosed. The cause is unknown; it is thought that it may be due to a virus. Most patients suffer slight damage to the nervous system; a few become severely paralysed.

Attacks have been said to have been precipitated by threats to security, death of a loved one, family conflicts, etc.

Hyperthyroidism

Hyperthyroidism is produced by an excessive secretion of thyroid hormones. The condition resembles an anxiety state. There is often a family incidence. Acute or prolonged stress can be precipitating and perpetuating factors.

Eczema and other skin diseases

Patients with atopic eczema develop itching, red and oedematous lesions on the skin, and attacks usually begin in early childhood and are liable to persist and recur. Patients with eczema are said to be tense, anxious and hypersensitive, and can react to stress by developing skin lesions.

Other skin diseases in which psychological factors may play a role are:

> perianal and perigenital
>   itching,
> urticaria,
> itching,
> rosacea,
> psoriasis.

Chapter 5 · Affective psychoses

The affective psychoses are those in which there is a marked and pathological change in mood, towards excessive sadness or excessive happiness. They are:

> manic-depressive psychosis,
> neurotic depression,
> reactive depression,
> secondary depression.

Manic-depressive psychosis

In this psychosis the patient shows periodic swings into mania or depression or both.

1. CAUSES

The causes are unknown. Biochemical abnormalities have been implicated. Sodium and water retention occur in mania and to a lesser degree in depression. Amines, chemical substances in brain cells, show variations, and these are thought to be a factor. There can be some hormonal variations. Genetic factors are important, and there is often a family history of manic-depressive attacks.

2. CONSTITUTION

Manic depressives are likely to be of pyknic build, i.e. to be short, fat people with big broad chests and abdomens.

3. PERSONALITY

Manic-depressives may be:
a. cyclothymic: varying from mild depression to mild mania and back again;
b. depressive: quiet, self-absorbed and pessimistic;
c. manic: cheerful, lively and sociable.

4. PRECIPITATING FACTORS

There may sometimes be a precipitating factor, such as a physical illness, but sometimes none is apparent.

5. CLINICAL FEATURES: DEPRESSION

In northern climates attacks of depression are much more common than attacks of mania. They occur in varying degrees of severity. The first attack can occur in childhood, but it usually occurs at between 20 and 30 years. Attacks can begin slowly or suddenly, and untreated are likely to last for weeks or months.

(a) *Mild depression*
The symptoms are slight and often physical. The patient may have fatigue, headache, numbness in the occipital region, vague abdominal pains, lack of energy, dryness of the throat; and if the true cause is unsuspected, he may undergo various investigations and treatments. He may be irritable, indecisive or aggressive. He is likely to express depressive ideas—that he has failed in life, that he has not lived up to promise, that he will never achieve anything worth while, that nothing is worth struggling for. He may not appreciate that he is ill. A woman may develop amenorrhoea.

(b) *Acute depression*
In this state the patient is severely depressed. The sort of ideas he expresses are that he is wicked, has done no good in the world, has achieved his position by fraud, deception or crime, and that his state is hopeless. He may believe that he is suffering from an incurable illness. He is likely to become suicidal. He may develop delusions of persecution, and may have auditory hallucinations of voices which abuse and threaten him. An acutely depressed man may murder his family and the family pets and then commit suicide, or a woman may murder her children.

Retardation is common, the patient having difficulty in thinking, and becoming slow in expressing his ideas and in all his activities. He sleeps badly and wakes in the early morning, at which time he is at his most depressed. Constipation, a slow pulse, a low blood pressure, and a dry mouth are common features.

(c) *Depressive stupor*
This is the severest form of depression. The patient is over-

whelmed by his depressive ideas and lies in stupor. He takes no notice of anything that is said to him, may not respond to painful stimuli, takes no food, and is likely to become dehydrated, constipated and retentive of urine.

6. CLINICAL FEATURES: MANIA ·

(a) *Hypomania*

This is the mildest degree of mania. The patient is very happy, tends to work too hard, takes on too much, tries to do other people's work, flits from task to task without completing any of them, and becomes a pest at home and at work. Usually he does not appreciate that there is anything wrong.

(b) *Acute mania*

The patient is elated and overactive; he talks incessantly, showing flight of ideas; he is regardless of ordinary decencies and conventions; he may be too excited to eat and drink, he sleeps badly if at all, and he can be destructive. Untreated the condition lasts for several weeks and is likely to end abruptly with a quick return to normality.

(c) *Delirious mania*

This very severe form of mania is uncommon. The patient becomes confused and delirious, can be very seriously ill, and can die.

Neurotic depression

In this depression there is usually a previous history of anxiety, hysterical reactions, or obsessional neurosis. There is often a precipitating factor, although it may be slight. The patient is anxious as well as depressed. His depression tends to get worse as the day goes on and he has difficulty in getting to sleep. He complains of various physical symptoms the severity of which varies from day to day. He is not mentally or physically retarded, and does not become deluded or hallucinated.

Reactive depression

This is a severe depression in a person of previously good health and mental stability who has become overwhelmed by severe misfortune.

Secondary depression

Depression can be a feature of some physical diseases and sometimes appears before other symptoms. These illnesses include:

carcinoma, of any organ,
cerebral tumour,
myxoedema,
alcoholism.

Influenza can be followed by severe depression.

PREVENTION OF MANIC AND DEPRESSIVE ILLNESSES

Lithium carbonate 250 mg twice daily is given to prevent manic and depressive illnesses in a person who is liable to have attacks of them.

TREATMENT OF DEPRESSION AND MANIA

1. *Mild depression*
The patient is usually looked after at home. Antidepressive drugs may be given, and he may require hypnotics at night if he is sleeping badly. He should give up work if it has become a burden to him, and other environmental stresses should if possible be relieved.

2. *Acute depression*
Because of the severity of the illness and the risk of suicide, the patient should be admitted to hospital and kept under observation. Active treatment is usually undertaken by:
a.   Antidepressive drugs, such as imipramine hydrochloride in doses of 75–150 mg daily in divided doses for patients under 60 and of up to 90 mg daily in divided doses for older patients; amitriptyline in doses of up to 225 mg daily in divided doses for patients under 60 and of up to 90 mg daily in divided doses for older patients; nortriptyline in doses of 20–100 mg daily in divided doses.

b. ECT: this is given for severe depression especially when accompanied by suicidal ideas, severe retardation and refusal to eat.

3. *Depressive stupor*
ECT is usually required to bring the patient out of stupor.

4. *Neurotic depression*
Treatment of neurotic depression is by supportive psychotherapy, removal if possible of environmental stresses, and tranquillizers or antidepressant drugs. Drugs of the MAOI group (monoamine oxidase inhibitors), such as phenelzine, iproniazid, and isocarboxazid, are said to be more effective for this kind of depression than other antidepressants.

5. *Reactive depression*
This is treated by one of the above methods according to the degree of depression.

6. *Hypomania*
Difficulties arise in the treatment of this condition because the patient may not regard himself as ill in any way. He should be persuaded to give up work, and be prescribed drugs such as haloperidol, chlorpromazine or lithium carbonate.

7. *Acute and delirious mania*
The patient has to be admitted to hospital. Care has to be taken that he receives adequate nourishment, and that his bowels and bladder are emptied. He may require protection from self-injury. His condition may respond to drug treatment by haloperidol, chlorpromazine or lithium carbonate. Treatment by ECT can stop an attack, and may be given if other methods fail.

Suicide

Suicide is common. The following factors are important.
1. *Mental illness.* Most suicides are suffering from a psychotic depression. Other conditions in which suicide can occur are early schizophrenia, alcoholism and psychopathy.
2. *Physical illness.* About a quarter of people who commit suicide are suffering from a severe physical illness.

3. *Age*. Old people are more likely to commit suicide than young and middle-aged people.
4. *Sex*. The incidence is higher in men than women.
5. *Social isolation*. People living alone are especially at risk.
6. *Method*. The commonest method is by drugs. Other methods are coal-gas poisoning (from car exhausts), hanging, drowning, shooting, stabbing, and burning.

Suicidal gestures

These gestures may be called attempted suicide, but they are often not intended to achieve suicide but to be an appeal for help by a person who is in an acute personal difficulty. The following factors are important.
1. *Sex*. The incidence is higher in women than in men.
2. *Age*. Adolescents or young adults.
3. *Family background*. They are usually the children of broken or unhappy homes.
4. *Social isolation*. The incidence is highest in unmarried, divorced or separated people. A partnership may have recently broken up.
5. *Drug abuse or alcoholism*. The patient is likely to be addicted to drugs or alcohol.
6. *Money*. There may have been a sudden loss of income.
7. *Number of attacks*. The patient may make several suicidal gestures.

Self-mutilation by wrist-slashing

A young woman inflicts multiple superficial cuts on her wrists, sometimes on other parts of the body, with a razor blade or piece of glass. The cuts are inflicted with a complete absence of pain.

PREVIOUS HISTORY

She is likely to have come from a broken home, to have suffered maternal deprivation in childhood, or to have been in hospital as a child. She may have been a nurse or have worked in paramedical employment. She may have had periods of over-eating or under-eating. The attack is likely to have been precipitated by parting from a person she is attached to, an acute personal problem, or threat of separation from a loved one. She may have seen someone else slash his or her wrists.

The wrist-slashing follows tension due to self-hatred, anger and acute depression, and the decision to do so may produce some relief.

TREATMENT

If suturing is necessary, it can be done without an anaesthetic for the patient is not likely to feel any pain in the slashed part. Psychiatric treatment is difficult. It is usually by tranquillizers, psychotherapy and attempts to relieve the patient's personal problems. The patient may have unpredictable mood-swings, and attempts to discharge her from hospital are likely to produce emotional storms and further attempts at self-mutilation.

Chapter 6 · Schizophrenia

Schizophrenia is a mental illness characterized by disturbance of normal thinking, a disturbance of emotion, a withdrawal from reality, abnormal behaviour of various kinds, and commonly delusions and hallucinations.

1. Incidence

The incidence of schizophrenia in European people is thought to be less than 1 per cent. It occurs in both sexes. Usually it begins in early adult life. It is rare in childhood, begins to be common in adolescence, has its maximum incidence at 18–35 years, and occurs less frequently in later life. Older patients are more likely to be women than men. It occurs more commonly among city dwellers than country dwellers, in people at the lower socioeconomic levels, and in immigrants than in natives of a country.

2. Causes

The causes of schizophrenia are not known. There may be more than one cause and several factors may act together to produce a similar clinical picture. Among the factors considered are the following.

(a) BIOCHEMICAL FACTORS

It is likely that some biochemical disorder of the brain interferes with normal cerebral functioning, but no definite factor has been identified.

(b) GENETIC FACTORS

The study of families and twins in which schizophrenia has occurred suggests that there is a genetic factor in some patients, who have inherited a liability to develop the condition.

(c) NEUROLOGICAL FACTORS

There is a higher incidence of abnormal EEGs (electro-encephalograms) than in the normal population, but these abnormalities are variable and non-specific.

(d) PRE-PSYCHOTIC PERSONALITY

About half the patients have had a schizoid pre-psychotic personality, one characterized by shyness, timidity, difficulty in making personal relationships, and a liability to think in abstract terms. But these features occur in people who do not develop schizophrenia, and the other half of patients with schizophrenia have shown no previous personality disorder.

(e) SOCIAL AND FAMILIAL FACTORS

A high proportion of schizophrenics come from the lower socioeconomic levels, but this is in part due to the downward drift of schizophrenics as their disease develops, recurs and incapacitates them. Family relationships may be abnormal. The father tends to be relatively weak and sometimes hostile to the patient; the mother tends to be dominant and overprotective; and both parents may minimize their child's abnormalities and deny that he or she is ill.

3. Clinical features

Schizophrenia may begin slowly, so slowly that it is not possible to say when it actually began, or suddenly and violently. There is considerable variation in clinical features, but the following are common.

(a) DETACHMENT FROM REALITY

In the early stages of a slow onset attack, the patient shows an increasing detachment from the normal world. He loses interest in ordinary affairs, from which he withdraws himself, and may come to be regarded as lazy. He may devote himself to the study of some abstract idea. At this stage a patient may develop an awareness that he is 'going mad' and this may drive him to attempt suicide; but in later stages all insight is lost.

Ideas of unreality are common. What he sees and hears are not quite what they should be. He looks at a face and it becomes distorted into unnatural and threatening shapes. Ideas of depersonalization may develop at the same time: he becomes doubtful about his own body, parts of which seem to be abnormal in peculiar ways; he may doubt which sex he belongs to.

(b) IDEAS OF REFERENCE AND PERSECUTORY DELUSIONS

The patient is liable to interpret in terms of himself anything he experiences. If his name happens to be Tomlinson, any mention of that name or any like it in the media, he interprets as referring to himself. If he sees the same man twice in the street he is being followed. From this develop delusions of persecution. Believing himself to be the victim of a plot, he is likely to think he is being poisoned, hypnotized, sterilized; he is followed wherever he goes; his house is bugged, his telephone is tapped. He may attribute his persecution to the man next door, to the police, to the Jews or the Arabs, to an international organization, the men from outer space. He may attack people he imagines are persecuting him. If the disease becomes chronic, he may develop grandiose delusions, such as that he is of royal blood or a TV star.

(c) HALLUCINATIONS

Hallucinations are commonly experienced. They are usually auditory. The patient hears threatening voices, endowed with an ultra-real quality. They may accuse him of being a murderer, a homosexual, a spy. Orders may be shouted at him so insistently that he must obey them. He may assault people from whom he believes these voices are coming.

Visual hallucinations occur less commonly: they are usually of faces or people or strange shapes. Hallucinations of smell, taste or touch are uncommon. The patient may think that his body smells in a peculiar way.

(d) EMOTIONAL CHANGES

Emotional changes are common from the onset of the disease. The patient becomes emotionally cold, loses his natural affections, shows no love for his family, no interest in it. A vicious resentment against one's relatives can develop.

(e) ABNORMAL BEHAVIOUR

The patient's behaviour can vary from normal to very abnormal. He usually withdraws from his normal activities, although some he may perform in a routine, stereotyped way. Apparently purposeless acts, peculiar gestures and mannerisms are common. There can be outbursts of violence and destruction or there can be apathy and stupor. He can show echolalia and echopraxia, automatic obedience, flexibilitas cerea, or negativism.

4. Types of schizophrenia

It is usual to describe the disease as occurring in various types, but these are not always clear-cut.

(a) SIMPLE SCHIZOPHRENIA

This begins in adolescence or early adult life. The patient withdraws himself from ordinary affairs to become preoccupied with vague hypochondriacal ideas or religious or philosophical problems. It is difficult to discover precisely what he is thinking about. His disorder of thought shows in a woolliness, a diffuseness of thinking, an inability to concentrate, a tendency to answer questions 'obliquely', i.e. slightly off the point. He is incapable of creative work, and if he works at all it is in some routine job which requires little thought, and he is likely to become unemployed and slip down the social scale. Delusions and hallucinations may not occur. Recovery is unlikely.

(b) HEBEPHRENIC AND CATATONIC SCHIZOPHRENIA

These two types are usually described separately, but they are very similar. Gross disturbances of behaviour occur in both. Attacks of excitement and violence can occur and alternate with gross apathy or stupor. Flexibilitas cerea, automatic obedience and negativism occur.

(c) PARANOID SCHIZOPHRENIA

This type of schizophrenia usually occurs in older patients. Its chief features are ideas of reference and delusions of persecution with complete absence of insight. Hallucinations, stupor, excitement and gross deterioration do not usually occur, and the patient's personality is well preserved.

(d) SCHIZO-AFFECTIVE SCHIZOPHRENIA

This type shows features of both schizophrenia and an affective psychosis, usually depression. There may be a definite precipitating factor and an acute onset.

(e) LATENT OR PSEUDO-NEUROTIC SCHIZOPHRENIA

In this type there are prominent 'neurotic' components of anxiety, obsessions and compulsions.

(f) CHRONIC SCHIZOPHRENIA

If chronicity develops, the patient lives in his abnormal thoughts, ordinary affairs mean little or nothing to him. Delusions are persecutory and grandiose. Hallucinations are common, and the patient responds to them by shouting or gesticulating. He may talk in a language of his own. Conduct may be stereotyped or unpredictable. Hoarding of rubbish and dressing or adorning oneself are common. The patient may bang or slap himself and attack other people. He can go on like this for years, eventually to die of some physical disease.

5. Prognosis

The course of the disease is variable and in the early days unpredictable. An attack can last for weeks, months, years or a lifetime. In general the more acute the disease the better the prognosis, but there are exceptions to this. The simple and paranoid types usually become chronic. Recovery from a first attack is, with modern treatment, common, but recovery after second and later attacks is less common, although rarely a chronic schizophrenic has recovered after years of illness.

6. Treatment

TREATMENT OF THE ACUTE PATIENT

(a) *General management*
The patient is admitted to a psychiatric hospital or to the psychiatric ward of a general hospital. If his behaviour is disturbed, he is likely to be nursed in a single room. He should so far as possible be kept under observation.

His food intake should be satisfactory. Feeding presents problems when the patient is disturbed or is deluded that the food is poisoned, and in severe cases the fluid and electrolyte balance is disturbed.

The nurse should be tolerant, patient and kind, and not easily upset by rebuffs and opposition. She should not go alone into a room when the patient might be dangerous, and she should not try to struggle single-handed with a patient; she should not turn her back on the patient or let him get between her and the door. She will have difficulty with the deluded patient who insists that she should agree with him. The nurse should not pretend to agree with ideas she knows are incorrect, nor must she strongly oppose them and point out how silly they are. The situation is a difficult one, and the nurse should try to persuade the patient that they agree to differ.

From the beginning the patient must be kept tidy and clean, and good personal habits must be insisted on. Supervision in bathing, shaving and dressing is often necessary.

(b) *Drugs*
Tranquillizers are often effective in controlling behaviour, reducing violence, abolishing or diminishing delusions and hallucinations, and shortening the time a patient has to spend in hospital. The ones in common use include:

chlorpromazine,	haloperidol,
trifluoperazine,	triperidol.

They are usually given by mouth, but in acute cases and when there is doubt whether the patient is taking them by mouth they can be given by intramuscular injection.

Hypnotics, such as paraldehyde and chloral hydrate, are sometimes necessary in addition to tranquillizers.

(c) *ECT*

ECT may be given for acute excitement, stupor, and when there is a strong depressive element in the illness.

(d) *Psychotherapy*

Psychotherapy may be given if the doctor believes that psychological factors are important in precipitating or maintaining the illness. It is given in single psychotherapeutic sessions or as group psychotherapy. Psychoanalysis is not thought to be of much avail and is not a standard treatment in Britain.

Behaviour therapy is used to replace unacceptable behaviour by acceptable behaviour.

(e) *Environmental therapy*

When a bad environment is thought to be a factor in the illness, the doctor or social worker attempts to improve it. This is likely to include counselling the family, and might involve the removal of the patient from an unsuitable home to a hostel. Rehabilitation programmes aim at adjusting the patient to live outside hospital and to work at a suitable job.

TREATMENT OF THE CHRONIC PATIENT

The chronic schizophrenic patient is likely to require care for life. He generally leads a routine life in which the nurse has to give attention to the maintenance of cleanliness, neat dress, adequate food intake and sleep. She should know her patient well enough to tell which peculiarities of behaviour are tolerable and which should be checked. She should be able to find in each patient some aspect of character which she can use for the patient's good. The good nurse continues to strive to find for each of her patients some approach, some interest and some understanding of the peculiar workings of the patient's mind by which he can be improved.

Behaviour therapy is used to improve behaviour.

Tranquillizers, given by mouth or intramuscular injection, improve the behaviour of many patients, and may enable them to live outside hospital. Regular administration is necessary, and relapse is likely to occur if the patient does not take the drug. ECT is occasionally necessary.

Paranoid states

A number of conditions occur in which delusions of persecution or grandeur are the predominant feature. Some psychiatrists consider them to be variants of schizophrenia and not separate conditions.

Paraphrenia is usually seen in women over the age of 40, who develop delusions of a very bizarre kind. They are totally devoid of insight and do not usually become hallucinated.

Paranoia is the development of a fixed delusion in a person who does not usually show any other sign of abnormality. A persecutory delusion of this kind may cause a patient to attack murderously the person he considers responsible.

Paranoid states in which delusions are expressed occur in senile dementia, in depression, and chronic alcoholism. Some deaf and blind people become paranoid as a reaction to their isolation.

The prognosis for these conditions is poor.

Chapter 7 · Psychopathic states

The term psychopathic state is not easy to define, for it is used to describe a number of conditions that do not fit into the ordinary pattern of neurotic or psychotic illness, although the patient may at times show features of either. A *psychopath* could be defined as a person who behaves in an irresponsible way and commits antisocial and sometimes aggressive acts regardless of their effects upon other people, and who is unaffected by any punishment he may suffer in consequence. An essential feature is that he has no feelings of shame or guilt, and does not alter his ways whatever is done for him or to him. He is liable to act impulsively, without consideration for others, and he may be liable to mood swings, of depression or elation, for little reason.

The condition is most apparent in the first half of adult life. As a child the psychopath may not have been noticeably abnormal, or he may have been regarded as cold and selfish, naughtier than other children, possibly a disturber of children's play, possibly cruel to insects and animals. Gross manifestations of abnormality appear in adolescence or early adult life. In middle age the more disturbed psychopath may improve and cease to be a problem. Some commit suicide.

Psychopathic behaviour takes many forms, varying with the degree of intelligence of the person, the degree of aggessiveness in his make-up, the kind of society he lives in, and the approximation of his condition to a neurosis or psychosis.

The intelligent psychopath and pathological liar

This kind of psychopath lives on his wits. He prefers not to follow an employment, he does not like work, and if he takes up a job he does not stick to it for long. To get money he sponges on relatives or women, blackmails, passes dud cheques, steals and sells stolen goods. He may be a man of considerable personal charm, well dressed, well spoken, plausible and immaculate.

He is often a pathological liar. He invents wonderful tales of his life, embellishing them with stories of military, diplomatic, financial and amorous triumphs, described in convincing detail. If he is caught out in a lie, he is not abashed and proceeds to tell a bigger one. He can be very fascinating to women and rapidly possesses their money and their person, and in spite of this a woman may remain devoted to him. He may give himself a title, wear a uniform and decorations he is not entitled to, put up at the best hotels, order expensive goods, and depart with the bills unpaid. His family may pay up to avoid a scandal; but there comes a time when his relatives disown him and he goes to prison. He may be sent to hospital for treatment, but there is nothing that can be done for him and he is not willing to stay. He may have mood swings, have vivid sexual phantasies and commit violent sex crimes. In lower walks of life the psychopath may live by stealing or scrounging, or on the earnings of prostitutes.

The aggressive psychopath

This psychopath is usually of low intelligence. He is moody, irritable, resentful and aggressive; he can attack people without provocation or for the slightest of reasons. At the times of these assaults his consciousness is impaired to some extent.

The electro-encephalogram (EEG) may be abnormal, with a persistence into adult life of slow waves, as if the brain were late in maturing; and a disappearance of these waves in middle life is associated with an improvement in his behaviour. Some tall aggressive psychopaths have a chromosome abnormality—they have 2 Y (male sex) chromosomes instead of one.

Treatment by tranquillizers and anticonvulsants may improve some of these patients.

Kleptomania

Kleptomania is a morbid impulse to steal. Most people who steal do so because they are short of money or food, have been taught to steal, enjoy stealing, or are overwhelmed by the display of goods in shops. Some steal during periods of stress. The psychopathic kleptomanic is usually a woman with plenty of money who repeatedly steals from shops, from the homes of friends, from fellow guests in hotels. The articles she steals may be of little value, and she may hoard them and never use them.

When caught the woman denies the offence, protests her innocence or offers a specious excuse. She is very likely to continue to repeat the offence.

Arsonists

An arsonist has an impulse to set fire to rubbish or buildings. He usually begins in a small way, and goes on to cause big fires. He may get sexual or other satisfaction from the sight of a fire or fire-brigade.

Eccentric psychopaths

These psychopaths behave, dress or talk in some eccentric way. They are often paranoid or paraphrenic. They may be solitary or they may gather around them other eccentric or unstable people, over whom they exercise considerable influence. They are founders of new religions, cults and societies. Some are litigious, write to the newspapers about their ideas, and abuse or threaten with legal action any one who expresses disbelief. Some progress to a schizophrenic psychosis.

Hysterical psychopaths

These psychopaths behave in a histrionic way. They over-react to a situation—with outbursts of noisy interest and affection, or with tears and recrimination. They are egocentric and over-dramatize situations. Some may be 'poison pen' writers.

Sexual psychopaths

This can take several forms. Sexual behaviour varies with differing cultures and societies, and some people may consider normal what others regard as abnormal.

Homosexuality is attraction towards persons of the same sex and sometimes physical relations with them. Fetishism is an association of sexual desire with some part of another's body, with underclothing or with some special fabric or object. Transvestism is the wearing of clothes normally worn by the other sex. Fetishists and transvestites may steal such clothing from shops or off washing-lines. Exhibitionsim is the exposure of the sexual organs to the opposite sex. Sadism is the derivation of sexual pleasure by inflicting pain on the sexual partner; masochism is the obtaining of pleasure from submitting to pain.

ı

Chapter 8 · Alcoholism

1. Definition

Alcoholism is present when a person cannot control his drinking, and when his drinking interferes with his personal relationships and socioeconomic functioning, or is producing mental and physical ill-health.

2. Alcohol

The alcohol in alcoholic drinks is ethyl alcohol. It is usually quickly absorbed from the stomach and small intestine, but absorption is delayed by the presence of food in the stomach. It is not stored in the body, and most of it is converted into carbon dioxide and water; a small amount is excreted as alcohol in the urine.

Alcohol depresses the control normally exercised by the cerebral cortex and so produces elation, talkativeness and excitement.

In chronic alcoholism a failure of absorption and utilization of the vitamin B group produces degeneration of nerve cells, to which are attributable some of the features of chronic alcoholism.

3. Incidence

Alcoholism is more common in men than women; with increased drinking by women and young people, the incidence in these groups is rising. There are thought to be about 300,000 chronic alcoholics in Britain, of whom about 80,000 are severely affected.

Alcoholism is an occupational hazard for:

> people in the drink trade (brewers, wine merchants, publicans),
> senior executives of firms (because of entertaining habits),
> commercial travellers (for the same reason),
> journalists,
> merchant navy sailors.

Vulnerable men are lonely widowers, divorcees and others living alone.

Women most likely to become alcoholics are:
professional women suffering executive strain,
wives of senior executives,
women living alone,
divorced women,
unmarried mothers with children and no male or family support.

The 'average alcoholic' begins to drink in youth, is drinking heavily and having drinking bouts by 26, experiences 'black-outs' at 30–35, and a few years later cannot control his drinking, has lost contact with his family, and is drinking alone.

4. Personality of alcoholics

Some alcoholics have unstable and inadequate personalities. Alcohol can be regarded as the means by which pleasant sensations are produced and unpleasant ideas and situations forgotten and avoided. Alcoholism may be an indication of an underlying neurosis or psychosis, or of psychotherapy. An anxiety-ridden person may drink to relieve his anxiety, and a manic-depressive may drink excessively when in mania or depression. Other conditions which can cause heavy drinking are epilepsy, early schizophrenia and head injury.

Psychoanalytically alcoholism is regarded as a wish to return to the mother's breast, or as an indication of hidden homosexuality, or as a drive towards self-destruction.

There may be a genetic factor contributing to alcoholism in men, but not necessarily in women. There is possibly an inherited biochemical predisposition to dependence on alcohol.

5. Clinical features of alcohol dependence

An alcoholic is likely to show psychological, behavioural and physical evidence of his condition.

(a) PSYCHOLOGICAL AND BEHAVIOURAL PATTERNS

The following patterns are likely to occur, not necessarily all in one person.

intellectual deterioration,
resentment and jealousy,
threats at suicide,
loss of family contact,
frequent motor accidents,
impairment of judgment,
delusions about spouse's fidelity,
frequent change of employment,
Monday morning absenteeism,
convictions for drunkenness and drunken driving.

(b) PHYSICAL ABNORMALITIES

The occurrence in one person of several of the following would suggest that he is an alcoholic:

flushed face,	breath smelling of drink,
bruises,	obesity,
black-outs,	tremor of lips and fingers,
dyspepsia,	unsteady gait.

6. Alcoholic diseases

(a) DIPSOMANIA

Dipsomania is an uncontrollable urge to drink excessively in bouts of a few days or weeks. Between bouts the person may drink little or nothing. Periodic drinking of this kind can be an indication of manic or depressive mood swings or of epilepsy.

(b) MANIA A POTU

Mania a potu is a condition in which a person becomes violent and confused after the consumption of only a small amount of alcohol.

(c) DELIRIUM TREMENS

Delirium tremens is an acute confusional state likely to occur after a bout of heavy drinking by a chronic alcoholic; it can be precipitated by a fracture, other accident, or a physical illness. It can be partly due to a failure to absorb and utilize vitamins of the vitamin B group.

Clinical features are:

confusion,	anxiety,
restlessness,	irritability,
insomnia,	acute fear,
slurred speech,	tremor of tongue and fingers,
fits,	misinterpretation of environment
	e.g. thinking spots are insects.

With treatment recovery is likely, but death can be due to a secondary infection, heart failure or self-injury.

(d) ALCOHOLIC HALLUCINOSIS

Alcoholic hallucinosis occurs as a complication of chronic alcoholism. The patient develops delusions of persecution and hallucinations of accusatory and persecutory voices, and in consequence he may arm himself and attack others. It runs a longer course than delirium tremens, and delusional ideas may persist after any excitement has died down. Recovery can occur, but recurrence is likely, and dementia may eventually develop.

(e) KORSAKOFF'S PSYCHOSIS

Korsakoff's psychosis occurs as a complication of chronic alcoholism or after delirium tremens. The essential features are a severe loss of memory, disorientation and confabulation (the patient giving an account of wholly imaginary events). His physical condition is likely to be poor and he may show evidence of vitamin B group deficiency.

A similar condition sometimes occurs in cerebral arteriosclerosis, in cerebral tumour, after subarachnoid haemorrhage, and after head injury.

(f) CHRONIC ALCOHOLISM

Chronic alcoholism has developed when drinking impairs the patient's mental and physical health, disrupts his social and working life, and cannot be controlled by him. By this time the patient is rarely sober for very long. Mental deterioration shows itself in loss of memory, carelessness, untidiness, disregard of the usual conventions of one's class, neglect of duties and responsibilities, inability to work at one's former level, emotional disturbances, untruthfulness, empty talk and boasting. Paranoid ideas can develop with dangerous intensity, being usually developed against the patient's spouse, who is accused of having lovers and who may be assaulted or killed. Depression, suicidal attempts, and dementia can occur. Physical conditions due to alcoholism are obesity, chronic conjunctivitis, chronic bronchitis, peripheral neuritis, chronic gastritis, cirrhosis of the liver, pancreatitis, and cardiovascular degeneration.

(g) MENTAL HANDICAP

Mental handicap and congenital abnormalities can occur in children born to alcoholic mothers.

7. Prevention of alcoholism

The methods of prevention of alcoholism are not very successful, and are likely to remain unsatisfactory until genetic discoveries lead to the pinpointing of individuals most at risk. Methods in use are:

> education of young people in the dangers of alcoholism,
> restriction of sales,
> high taxation.

8. Treatment

(a) GENERAL

The treatment of the chronic alcoholic is difficult and often disappointing. Few patients will submit themselves to a life-long abstinence in a world where the inducements and temptations to drink are all around them. Occasionally a man or woman will come for help when jolted by a conviction for drunkenness or drunken driving; but if treatment is to succeed the alcoholic must have a genuine desire to be cured and be willing and able to change his job if it is one in which drinking is traditional. The doctor and nurse must be prepared to spend much time in supportive therapy, and the patient's nearest relatives must be prepared to become teetotal themselves so that there is no drink in the home and no parties in a pub.

Psychotherapy can be employed in an attempt to identify the causes of anxiety and relieve it. Lithium can be given to relieve depression.

Antabuse and Abstem are drugs which in combination with alcohol produce unpleasant symptoms such as nausea, vomiting and flushing of the face. The patient takes a tablet of it in the morning with the knowledge that if he takes alcohol during the day he will develop these symptoms.

Patients willing to be cured but unable to make the effort by themselves should be put into touch with Alcoholics Anonymous (number in local telephone directory), an organization of ex-alcoholics pledged to help alcoholics.

Hospital care is required for severe chronic alcoholics and for acute alcoholic illnesses. A hostel may be available to take the homeless, deteriorating alcoholic.

(b) TREATMENT OF ACUTE ALCOHOLIC ILLNESS

Treatment of delirium tremens and acute alcoholic hallucinosis is by:

> hospitalization,
> vitamin B preparations by intramuscular or intravenous injection,
> tranquillizers, such as diazepam (Valium) or haloperidol (Serenace, Haldol),
> correction of fluid and electrolyte imbalance,
> adequate food intake.

Chapter 9 · Drug addiction

A drug addict is a person who takes excessive amounts of a drug or drugs for prolonged periods and without medical indications, develops tolerance, and shows symptoms of withdrawal if he cannot get the drug.

Most addicts have shown abnormal, psychopathic traits before becoming addicted, and it is unusual for a mentally normal person to become an addict, except possibly to barbiturates. Any drug with sedative, stimulating or hallucinogenic properties can become a drug of addiction, and commonly a drug used to relieve the symptoms produced by withdrawal of another drug becomes itself liable to be a drug of addiction. In some parts of the world drugs may be taken daily in small amounts by large numbers of people—opium in the Far East, cocaine in South America, cannabis in Africa and Asia—and produce a mild addiction.

Drug dependence is the mental and physical state which develops between the addict and the drug. With drugs of addiction this shows itself in behavioural and other responses and in a compulsion to take the drug, both to appreciate its pleasurable effects and to avoid any unpleasantness that is produced by not taking it.

Drugs commonly used as drugs of addiction can be classified as:

> drugs that have a depressant effect,
> drugs that have a stimulant effect,
> drugs liable to produce hallucinations.

1. Drugs that have a depressant effect

BARBITURATES

Barbiturates are commonly prescribed for their sedative and hypnotic effect although better drugs are now available. Addiction is usually mild. Patients are liable to develop a dependence on the drug and to show symptoms when it is withdrawn. Tolerance of it has developed when the patient can take it without becoming sleepy. Features of dependence are:

dizziness,	tremor,
nausea,	postural hypotension,
ataxia,	irritability.

Withdrawal of the drug is liable to produce anxiety, tremor, sweating, palpitations and insomnia. Sudden withdrawal after large doses have been taken can produce a major epileptic fit.

MORPHINE

Addiction to morphine is most likely in those who have access to it—doctors, nurses and pharmacists. It is liable to produce:

loss of efficiency,
neglect of appearance,
disregard of social conventions,
rambling remarks,
sudden changes of mood,
decline in physical health—anaemia, constipation, low resistance to infection.

Withdrawal effects include nausea, vomiting, headache, anxiety, depression, insomnia, muscular cramps, sneezing, yawning, crying.

HEROIN

Heroin (diamorphine hydrochloride) easily produces addiction. It may be preferred to morphine because of the intensity of the euphoria it produces and the absence of the vomiting and constipation likely to be produced by morphine. Symptoms of addiction are similar to those of morphine addiction. Severe mental and physical deterioration occurs, and the addict is likely to die young—of sepsis, pneumonia, or pulmonary oedema.

2. Drugs that have a stimulating effect

AMPHETAMINE

Amphetamine and amphetamine-like drugs produce an addiction characterized by:

euphoria,   restlessness,

insomnia,
psychotic reactions with delusions of
    persecution and hallucinations,
excitement,

over-activity,
exhaustion,
aplastic anaemia.

Withdrawal produces anxiety, restlessness and insomnia.

COCAINE

Cocaine is usually taken by injection, but it can be sniffed up the nose (where it is liable to produce ulceration of the mucous membrane). It may be taken by morphine and heroin addicts to counteract the depressive effects of these drugs. It is likely to produce:

elation,
freedom from fatigue,
glibness,
short psychoses with confusion,
    delusions and hallucinations,

overactivity,
facile thoughts,
restlessness.

Cocaine addicts are often gross psychopaths, alcoholics, multiple-drug takers, female or male prostitutes; and treatment is usually unsuccessful.

3. Drugs liable to produce hallucinations

CANNABIS

Cannabis can produce acute or chronic reactions. An acute reaction is usually dose-related, but a novice may get one after smoking a single cigarette. Features are:

ideas of depersonalization,
delusions,
confusion,
excitement,
delirium,

paranoid ideas,
hallucinations,
restlessness,
severe panic,
disorientation.

Chronic reactions are apathy, indifference to current affairs, decline in observance of social conventions, and a deterioration in behaviour. A short paranoid psychosis can occur.

    Addiction to cannabis may not cause severe antisocial behaviour. Some addicts can give it up spontaneously and others continue to take it indefinitely. Its particular danger is that it can lead to taking more dangerous hallucinogenic drugs such as LSD.

LSD

LSD (lysergic acid diethylamide) is a hallucinogenic drug more dangerous than cannabis. It produces:

    a dream-like state,
    disorders or perception,
    hallucinations,
    emotional disturbances,
    loss of control of behaviour leading to violence, murder, and
      suicide.

Chronic addiction causes apathy and mental deterioration.

Treatment of drug addiction

There is no satisfactory treatment for drug addiction. Success can be expected only if the patient is fully willing to cooperate and desirous of a cure. Treatment is carried out by gradual withdrawal of the drug with, for a time, substitution by other, less harmful drugs during the period of withdrawal, which is often disturbed and stormy. Modified insulin treatment may be tried. Some form of psychotherapy may be attempted. Relapse is very common.

Chapter 10 · Psychiatric results of brain injury

In severe injuries the substance of the brain is torn and massive haemorrhages can occur in it or the extradural space, or multiple small haemorrhages can occur in the brain substance; cerebral oedema can occur, and nerve fibres can in time lose their myelin sheaths and become incapable of transmitting impulses. But the nature of the change that produces concussion is obscure. It is able to produce an immediate disturbance of cerebral function, and there may be degeneration of nerve fibres without apparent damage to brain cells or interference with their blood supply.

Concussion

In concussion an immediate loss of consciousness is associated with muscular paralysis. It can be slight, moderate or severe.

In *slight concussion* there may be an incomplete loss of consciousness or complete loss of consciousness lasting from a few seconds to a few hours. It can be followed by confusion, headache and drowsiness.

In *moderate concussion* the patient is unconscious for several hours and emerges slowly from it. For hours or days afterwards he shows clouding of consciousness, irrational thought processes, disorientation in time and place, confabulation, misidentification of people and of events. He may develop acute delirium with delusions, hallucinations, excitement and possibly violence; after that he can pass into a state of apathy with gross loss of memory.

In *severe concussion* the patient is unconscious for days or weeks, is severely shocked, and can die. Delirium and other gross disturbances are to be expected in those who recover consciousness.

Retrograde amnesia is common after concussion: it is a loss of memory for the event that caused the concussion and sometimes for events immediately before it. A man remembers riding his motor-cycle but not hitting a car; the footballer remembers playing football but not the kick that laid him out. The more severe the concussion the longer the amnesia is likely to be for, but it gradually shrinks except in demented patients.

Post-traumatic amnesia is the period of time from the injury until the patient is continuously aware of his surroundings, and the length of this time is a measure of both the severity of the concussion and the length of time the patient is likely to be off work.

Post-concussional syndrome

The actuality of a post-concussional syndrome has been doubted for it is thought to occur only in people with a neurotic pattern of behaviour or who have had definite neuroses; and it is considered that the symptoms can only be attributed to the injury if there are neurological signs of disease or an abnormal electroencephalogram (EEG). Likely symptoms are a chronic throbbing headache, giddiness on change of posture, anxiety, difficulty in concentrating, blackouts, fluctuating moods, irritability, insomnia, fatigue and intolerance of noise. A prospect of receiving compensation may be a strong factor in maintaining the condition.

A *fugue state*, in which the patient wanders away from home in a state of impaired consciousness and is subsequently unable to account for his movements and actions, can occur after brain injury in a person with a hysterical or psychopathic personality.

A post-concussional syndrome has been described in children, but the presence and intensity of the symptoms are dependent not so much upon the severity of the injury as upon the child's previous personality and the personalities of his parents. The symptoms are usually nervousness, anxiety, lack of concentration, irritability, bad temper, overactivity, decline in school work, enuresis, aggressiveness and antisocial behaviour.

Post-traumatic epilepsy

Epilepsy occurs in 2–4 per cent of brain injuries. Fits usually occur within 2 years of the injury, but can occur much later. Those that occur within a few days of the injury usually stop spontaneously, and the longer the interval between the injury and the occurrence of the first fit the more likely is the epilepsy to persist. Children are more likely to develop fits than adults. Major fits are the most common, but other kinds can occur.

Post-traumatic dementia

Post-traumatic dementia is especially likely to occur in patients after severe concussion, and a prolonged delirum, and in old people and arterio-sclerotics. Old people hardly ever recover completely from severe concussion.

The dementia is due either to extensive destruction of nerve cells and tracts, or to a catastrophic disturbance of cerebral functioning without apparent destruction of nerve tissue.

The patient does not return to normal after the injury. He continues to show such symptoms as inability to concentrate, difficulty in studying, loss of memory, poor association of ideas, poverty of ideas and a reduction in reasoning power. Degenerative changes in the prefrontal lobes of the brain are liable to produce moodiness, irritability, explosive mood changes, irresponsibility and outbursts of violence. Symptoms of this kind persisting over 18 months are very likely not to improve, and the prognosis for a patient with post-traumatic dementia is bad.

Punch-drunkenness is a post-traumatic dementia produced in boxers by blows to the head or hitting the head on the floor of the ring. Typical features are loss of memory, decline in intelligence, slowness, dullness, fatuousness, slurred speech, ataxia, coarse tremor of the hands, abnormal jealousy, and outbursts of rage and violence. The prognosis is bad.

Chronic subdural haematoma

A chronic subdural haematoma is due to bleeding into the subdural space. An apparently trivial injury may be sufficient to produce the bleeding, which may be slow and not produce symptoms for several weeks or months after the injury. Most patients with it are over the age of 70.

Symptoms are headache, drowsiness, apathy or excitement, confusion, fits and irresponsible behaviour. Very typically the symptoms vary in occurrence and severity from day to day. A Korsakoff's psychosis can occur.

The patient may show no neurological evidence of disease, but papilloedema (swelling of the optic discs, visible on ophthalmoscopic examination) can be present. The cerebrospinal fluid (CSF) can be normal, or be yellow, under increased pressure or with an increased protein content. Encephalography may show the presence of a space-occupying lesion, and the electro-encephalogram (EEG) may be abnormal. Treatment is by surgical removal of the haematoma either through a burr hole or by open operation.

Psychosis

A psychosis of a schizophrenic, paranoid, or manic-depressive kind can occur after a brain injury, but only rarely can be attributed to it. Almost all patients who have developed a psychosis after brain injury have had previous attacks or had an abnormal personality before the event.

Psychiatric treatment

Treatment should begin as soon as the patient recovers consciousness. In addition to his uncertain hold on consciousness, confusion and headache, he will be bewildered by what has happened to him. He has to be told simply what has happened to him, the information being repeated many times over hours or days, for he will have difficulty in grasping it and remembering it. From the first he must be surrounded by positive optimism, he must be reassured over and over again that he will recover, and he must not be asked for symptoms he might have unless he first complains of them himself.

He must be got out of bed as soon as he is fit to and be engaged in exercises, games, occupational therapy and work designed to give him reassurance and promote a return to his former skills. Treatment of an acute neurosis may be necessary. Drugs should be avoided as they are liable to cause apathy or addiction.

Chapter 11 · Neurosyphilis

Neurosyphilis is the term used to describe the diseases produced by the infection of the nervous system with the *treponema pallidum*, the micro-organism that causes syphilis.

Infection of the nervous system and its meninges and blood vessels takes place during the primary and secondary stages of syphilis. Some patients show no evidence of this invasion; others have malaise, headache, irritability, spinal pains and occasionally confusion or delirium, with the cerebrospinal fluid (CSF) being under increased pressure and with an increase of the amount of protein and number of cells in it. Tissue reactions then subside, the organisms may be destroyed, and the patient feels better. In a number of cases the organism is not destroyed, but remains in the nervous tissue for several years without causing symptoms. With the passage of years the patient's resistance to the disease can diminish and the organisms then become active again and produce evidence of disease during the tertiary stage of syphilis.

Asymptomatic syphilis is syphilis during the quiescent period. The only sign of syphilis at this time can be an Argyll-Robertson pupil, which is small, irregular and not reacting to light. The CSF may be abnormal, showing an increased number of cells, increased protein content, a positive Wassermann Reaction (WR), or an abnormal Lange curve.

Meningovascular syphilis

In menigovascular syphilis the blood vessels and meninges of the nervous system are primarily affected. Inflammatory changes take place in them and cause a reduction in the blood supply to the nervous tissue.

CLINICAL FEATURES

It develops usually between 3 months and 5 years after the primary infection. The onset is rapid. Symptoms and signs are variable and liable to fluctuation. They include:

malaise,	fatigue,
headache,	dizziness,
fits,	cranial nerve paralysis,
hemiplegia,	aphasia,
apraxia,	confusion,
delirium,	sphincter disturbance.

SPECIAL TESTS

WR and other tests for syphilis in the blood are usually positive. CSF shows increased pressure, increased number of cells, increased amount of protein, usually a positive WR, and an abnormal Lange curve.

TREATMENT

Penicillin is given intramuscularly in doses of 1 million units daily for 12–15 days. On recovery the patient may be left with some permanent damage to the nervous system.

General paralysis of the insane

General paralysis of the insane (GPI) is a chronic syphilitic infection of the nervous system, producing a progressive dementia and paralysis. It occurs usually between the ages of 30 and 50 years. It occurs in about 5 per cent or less of all people infected with syphilis, and there may be a special strain of the organism that has a particular affinity for nervous tissue.

The cells of the cortex of the brain degenerate and die, and the brain atrophies in consequence. The meninges become thickened and adherent to the brain. Blood-vessels are little affected. The organism can be found in affected nervous tissue.

CLINICAL FEATURES

The disease can develop slowly over several months or quickly over a few days. Its course is described in three phases—early, middle, and late. The middle and late phases will not develop if the disease is adequately treated in the early phase.

Early phase

> early signs of dementia, with forgetfulness, irresponsibility,
>   inability to express thoughts clearly,
> depression or euphoria or emotional instability,
> headache,
> loss of weight,
> fits,
> loss of muscle tone,
> tremor, slurred speech,
> pupil abnormalities,
> tendon reflex abnormalities.

Middle phase

> severe dementia,
> depression or elation with delusions of grandeur,
> delusions of persecution,
> fits,
> hallucinations,
> hemiparesis,
> difficulties in speaking, standing, walking,
> exaggerated tendon reflexes,
> extensor plantar reflexes.

Late phase

> gross dementia,
> fits,
> loss of sphincter control,
> emaciation,
> bedsores,
> secondary infection,
> death.

SPECIAL TESTS

Blood: WR usually positive. CSF: increased cells, increased protein, WR positive, abnormal Lange curve.

TREATMENT

After a day of small doses to detect unusual responses, penicillin is given in daily doses of 600,000–1 million units until 12 million units have been given. This should be enough to abolish symptoms and achieve a cure. Progress is checked by examination of the CSF, and especially of its cell count, which in a cured patient should return to normal. The CSF is examined at 6-monthly intervals for a year, and then once a year for 5 years. If there are any signs of recurrence (which shows first in an increase in the number of cells in the CSF), another course of penicillin is given, and the patient's progress monitored.

Tabes dorsalis

Tabes dorsalis (locomotor ataxia) is a chronic syphilitic disease of the spinal cord, spinal nerves and cranial nerves. It occurs in less than 5 per cent of people who have had syphilis, and usually occurs 15–25 years after the primary infection. More men are affected than women.

CLINICAL FEATURES

The course of the disease is slowly progressive over years. Symptoms and signs are variable and numerous:

> lightning pains in the limbs—sudden recurrent attacks of severe shooting or stabbing pains in various places in the limbs,
>
> visceral crises—acute pain and disorder of function in the stomach, rectum or bladder,
>
> heaviness or numbness in the limbs,
>
> ataxia,
>
> impotence,
>
> rombergism—an inability to stand without swaying when the feet are together and the eyes shut,
>
> cranial nerve paralysis,
>
> optic atrophy, blindness,
>
> loss of sphincter control,
>
> perforating ulcer of feet,
>
> Charcot joint—joint is painlessly enlarged and grossly disorganized.

Tabo-paresis shows features of both GPI and tabes dorsalis. It runs a chronic course with a simple dementia.

TREATMENT

Courses of penicillin are given. Damage to the nervous system is likely to be persistent. Tabetic pains are treated by pain-removing drugs; morphine or pethidine may be necessary.

Congenital syphilis

Where treatment of syphilis is good and there is good antenatal care, congenital syphilis does not occur. It can cause mental handicap and rarely a congenital form of general paralysis.

Chapter 12 · Epilepsy

The term epilepsy is used to describe sudden loss of consciousness, often associated with convulsions or convulsive phenomena. Epilepsy is not a disease in itself, but an expression of abnormal cerebral functioning, arising from any one of a number of causes. These causes may be local conditions in the brain or general diseases of the body. The word epilepsy means a seizure; the words fit, convulsion, and seizure all mean the same.

Primary or idiopathic epilepsy is epilepsy for which no physical cause can be found. It is thought to be due to an abnormality of cerebral physiology, in which several genetic factors are involved.

Secondary epilepsy is epilepsy for which a definite physical cause can be demonstrated. Among the causes are:

> congenital disease or deformity of the brain,
> anoxia (lack of oxygen) during birth,
> injury of the brain,
> encephalitis, meningitis, syphilis of the brain,
> tumour, abscess or parasites in the brain,
> cerebrovascular disease: thrombosis, haemorrhage, embolism,
> any degeneration of the brain, dementia,
> uraemia,
> low blood sugar,
> heart block,
> hyperventilation causing alkalosis,
> poisoning by lead, carbon monoxide, alcohol,
> hydration due to excessive beer drinking,
> some drugs: bemigride, leptazol, barbiturate intoxication.

Reflex epilepsy is epilepsy produced by the rapid repetition of a stimulus, such as a flashing light. Watching and hearing a train go by or adjusting a flickering TV set can produce epilepsy in some people by provoking an EEG abnormality.

Incidence

About 1 person in 200 has a fit at some time in his life. Epilepsy occurs equally in both sexes. About 1 patient in 3 has his first fit before the age of 10, and about 2 in 3 before 30. Some children have so unstable a nervous system that they have fits during fevers, teething or irritation by worms; a few continue to have fits later. If one parent is epileptic, the incidence of epilepsy or psychopathy in his or her children is about 10–15 per cent and of epilepsy alone about 6 per cent. If both parents are epileptic or one is epileptic and the other has an abnormal EEG, the incidence is higher.

Electro-encephalogram

An abnormal electro-encephalogram (EEG) is usually present in epilepsy, although some epileptics have a normal EEG and some people who have never had a fit have an abnormal EEG.

A fit is the product of an abnormal discharge from neurones in the brain. Two types of abnormal wave are common:

a. a violent discharge of abnormally fast or abnormally slow waves during a major fit;

b. a pattern of alternating spikes and waves during a minor fit.

Abnormal waves of various kinds can be present between fits.

In major and minor fits the abnormal discharge is thought to originate in the reticular formation (the centrally situated part of the brain concerned with consciousness) and to spread from it into the cerebral hemispheres. In other fits the discharge does not spread so extensively and does not produce unconsciousness. In jacksonian epilepsy the discharge begins in or just beneath the cerebral cortex, and consciousness is not lost unless the discharge spreads into the reticular formation.

Types of fit

There are several types of fit. Some patients have only one type of fit; others have fits of several types.

MAJOR FIT

The characteristics of a major fit are as follows.

1. A *prodromal period* sometimes; the patient is irritable for several hours or days before the fit occurs.

2. An *aura* occasionally precedes loss of consciousness; the patient feels that something is going to happen; his muscles twitch or he experiences a peculiar smell or taste.

3. The *tonic* stage begins. The patient loses consciousness suddenly and completely. If he is standing he falls to the ground. He may utter a short, dry sound as he loses consciousness. Then he develops muscular rigidity with arms and legs in extension. His jaw is clenched and if his tongue protrudes it is liable to be bitten. The eyeballs roll upwards. Respiration ceases, cyanosis appears, there is frothing from the mouth and the froth may be blood-stained. The bladder and sometimes the bowel are emptied. This state lasts for 30–60 seconds.

4. The *clonic stage* then develops. The patient remains unconscious. Muscular rigidity is replaced by alternate muscular contractions and relaxations, with jerking of head, trunk and limbs. Breathing is resumed noisily. Perspiration breaks out all over the body. The tongue may be bitten again. This stage lasts for 1–5 minutes.

5. *State of recovery.* Consciousness returns and muscular contractions cease. The patient may complain of headache or be confused. Pyrexia, speech disturbances, albuminuria and muscular pains may occur. *Post-epileptic automatism* sometimes occurs: the patient performs some apparently purposeful but inappropriate act, such as undressing, and he can get into trouble if he behaves like this in a public place; his behaviour may be seriously disturbed, and he may even attack people.

MINOR FIT

The characteristic feature of this kind of epilepsy is a momentary loss of consciousness. It is also called an 'absence' or a 'lapse attack'. Its characteristics are as follows.

1. The patient loses consciousness suddenly and for a few seconds.

2. He stops what he is doing and drops anything he is holding; he may go pale or have slight twitching of face and fingers.

3. He does not convulse or wet himself.

4. On recovery of consciousness he goes on with what he was doing before.

Minor fits begin in childhood or adolescence. Single or multiple attacks occur. Some patients have 100 or more attacks in a day. The patient may also have major fits.

TEMPORAL LOBE EPILEPSY

This is produced by lesions in one or both temporal lobes and has characteristics of its own. It can begin at any age. The characteristics are these.

1. Symptoms are varied.
2. Peculiar experiences of smell, taste, sight and hearing can occur.
3. Impairment of consciousness, disorientation, dream-states and disturbances of memory can occur.
4. Movements of tongue and lips, wandering or running about and violence can occur.

JACKSONIAN EPILEPSY

This kind of fit is named after Hughlings Jackson, a British neurologist, who described it. It is produced in the cortex of the cerebrum, the part where it begins being called the 'trigger area'. Motor or sensory fits can occur.

A *motor fit* is characterized by muscular contractions which begin in one part of the body—usually a thumb, a big toe or a corner of the mouth—whence they can spread to other parts in accordance with their representation in the cerebral cortex. The contractions can stop at any stage. Consciousness is not lost unless the impulse spreads to a deeper part of the brain, when a major fit can develop.

A *sensory fit* is characterized by abnormal sensations beginning in one part of the body and spreading to other parts. Consciousness is not lost.

MYOCLONIC EPILEPSY

This kind of epilepsy is characterized by slight muscular twitching without loss of consciousness. It is sometimes associated with major fits or akinetic epilepsy.

AKINETIC EPILEPSY

This kind of epilepsy is characterized by a sudden loss of muscle tone, the patient falling to the ground without losing consciousness. It can be associated with other kinds of epilepsy.

STATUS EPILEPTICUS

This is the condition in which one fit succeeds another without the patient regaining consciousness between them. The number of fits varies from a few to several thousand, and the period of unconsciousness can last from an hour to several days. It is not uncommon in severe, chronic epileptics. It is usual to attribute them to stopping an anticonvulsant drug too suddenly or to the onset of infection, but in many cases there is no discernible cause. Most attacks stop spontaneously or with treatment. Death can occur from heart failure or pulmonary complications.

Course

The course of epilepsy is variable. Some patients have only one fit a year or more rarely; others have several in a day and hundreds in the course of the year. A succession of fits may be followed by freedom from them for weeks or months. Some patients have fits only at night (nocturnal epilepsy). Spontaneous remission can occur at any time and last for years or for life, and freedom from fits can be produced by drugs. Death in or just after a fit can occur.

Mental condition

Some epileptics are of average or above-average intelligence. But epilepsy is common among the mentally handicapped, and there are more epileptic children below than above average intelligence.

Infrequent fits and minor fits do not appear to affect intelligence, but a patient who has a lot of major fits is liable to develop deterioration of intelligence and personality. The severe chronic epileptic is likely to be irritable, moody, egocentric, hypochondriacal and suspicious. He may have outbursts of temper and violence and also delusions of persecution and hallucinations, usually of voices. The degeneration may be due to a combination of having fits, taking anticonvulsant drugs, and being rejected by society, for an epileptic is commonly shunned by people who know he has fits, and he often has difficulty in obtaining and holding a job, and in consequence he is likely to become sullen and embittered.

Treatment

DRUGS

The aim of drug treatment in epilepsy is the achievement of the maximum anticonvulsant effect with the minimum of side effects; and the correct doses for an individual are those that can do this for him. Effective control may be achieved by one drug or by several in combination. Except when toxic effects are being produced, no drug is stopped suddenly because of the danger of increasing the number of fits or possibly precipitating an attack of status epilepticus; any change should be spread over a fortnight, the dose of the old drug being reduced as the dose of the new drug is increased.

Anticonvulsants must be taken regularly and no dose should be omitted. The responsibility of taking the right dose at the right time usually rests upon the patient, but if the patient is a child or unfit to take the responsibility, it should rest with one relative and not with several. Parents and relatives should be impressed with the importance of regular administration, of honesty in admitting any omission or overdose, and of observation of any complication. The patient should not allow himself to run out of drugs. Anticonvulsants do not usually need to be taken more often than twice a day. To help the patient who may forget whether he has taken a dose or not, he should put the daily dose into a little bottle labelled with the day of the week. He can then check if he has taken the right amount on the right day.

Drug concentrations in the blood can be measured and related to the incidence of fits and complications.

Drugs commonly used are listed below.

1. For major fits, temporal lobe epilepsy, jacksonian epilepsy:
   phenobarbitone,
   phenytoin sodium,
   primidone,
   sulthiame,
   sodium valproate.

2. For minor fits:
    ethosuximide,
    troxidone,
    paramethadione.

Phenobarbitone
Dose:
    adults: 30–120 mg daily in divided doses;
    children up to 1 year 15–30 mg daily;
    children 1–5 years: 30–60 mg daily;
    children over 5: as for adults.

Phenobarbitone is still the usual drug of first choice for major fits in adults; it is less effective for temporal lobe and jacksonian epilepsy. It is suspected of causing aggressive behaviour and other behaviour problems in children.
    Toxic effects: drowsiness, blurring of vision.

Phenytoin sodium (Epanutin, Dilantin)
Dose: 50–200 mg daily in divided doses.
It increases the number of minor fits.
    Toxic effects: hypertrophy of gums, gastric upsets, excessive growth of hair on face and limbs, allergic reactions, cerebellar syndrome (giddiness, ataxia, nystagmus).

Primidone (Mysoline)
Dose: 500 mg–2 g daily in divided doses.
It is probably less effective than phenobarbitone.
    Toxic effects: drowsiness, giddiness, vomiting, ataxia, confusion, megaloblastic anaemia.

Sulthiame (Ospolot)
Dose: 100–600 mg daily in divided doses.
Some patients respond well to it, some show little or no improvement.
    Toxic effects: gastrointestinal upsets, tingling in extremities, breathlessness, drowsiness, ataxia, confusion, depressive or schizophrenic psychosis, difficulty in swallowing, vomiting, renal damage.

Sodium valproate (Epilim)
Dose:

> adults: 400 mg–1.2 g daily in divided doses;
> children under 3: 20–30 mg per kilo per day;
> children 3–15 years: from 400 mg daily.

It can be also used for minor and temporal lobe epilepsy, and is a drug of first choice for children.

Toxic effects: drowsiness, nausea, loss or increase of appetite.

Ethosuximide (Zarontin, Emeside)
Dose:

> adults: up to 1 g daily in divided doses;
> children under 6: up to 250 mg daily in divided doses;
> children 6–12: up to 500 mg daily in divided doses.

It increases the number of major fits, and if the patient has both kinds, it is given with a drug effective against major fits.

Toxic effects: gastric upsets; rarely damages liver, kidney, bone marrow.

Troxidone (Tridione)
Dose:

> adults: 900 mg–1.8 g daily in divided doses;
> children: 300–900 mg daily in divided doses.

It can increase the number of major fits and is more toxic than ethosuximide.

Toxic effects: glare phenomenon (illuminated objects glitter like snow in sunshine), drowsiness, gastric disturbances, dermatitis, aplastic anaemia, renal damage, baldness.

Paramethadione (Paradione)
Dose:

> adults: 900 mg–1.8 g daily in divided doses;
> children: 300–900 mg daily in divided doses.

It is tried when other drugs are ineffective.
Toxic effects: similar to those of troxidone.

SURGERY

Small lesions of the brain that are producing fits can sometimes be localized by EEG and other investigations and removed surgically.

Such lesions are scar tissue, depressed fractures, bullets, cysts, encapsulated abscesses, encapsulated haemorrhages.

Hemispherectomy has been performed early in life for cerebral palsy associated with hemiplegia and fits; it can reduce the number of fits and improve behaviour. Dividing the corpus callosum (the thick band of fibres connecting the two cerebral hemispheres) is sometimes performed for severe, intractable epilepsy.

General care

CHILDHOOD

About 60,000 schoolchildren in Britain have epilepsy. Most of them are educated in ordinary schools. Learning and behaviour problems are more common in them than in normal children. Behavioural problems are greater in epileptic boys than epileptic girls. Common problems are learning difficulty, inattentiveness, drowsiness, emotional dependence and overactivity. For many children the drugs used to control epilepsy cause more problems than their fits; aggressiveness may be due to phenobarbitone, poor reading may be due to phenytoin sodium.

An epileptic child should be encouraged to lead as normal a life as possible and should if possible live at home. Children with severe epilepsy or severe behaviour disorders are admitted to special residential schools or are taught at home by a home teacher.

ADULT LIFE

Some kinds of work are unsuitable for an epileptic whose fits are not completely controlled—and it is impossible to guarantee that a controlled epileptic will not occasionally have a fit. The patient should not put himself or fellow workers in danger if he has a fit and should work where he can get help if he has a fit. Unsuitable work includes:

> driving a vehicle,
> working with machinery in which a person might be trapped,
> working where there is a risk of being burned or falling off a ladder,
> working in isolated places away from help.

Suitable work varies with the person's intelligence, aptitudes, physical build, and the frequency and severity of his fits. Suitable work includes:

assembly work in factories,	clerical work,
librarianship,	accountancy,
gardening,	handicrafts.
labouring,	

In spite of provisions for the employment of handicapped people, many firms are unwilling to employ epileptics and many workmen are unwilling to work with them, although where suitable precautions are taken their accident rate is no higher than that of non-epileptic people.

Epileptic colonies provide a home and work for epileptics whose fits are too frequent for them to live at home and work in ordinary employment.

Precautions

Wherever an epileptic is, certain precautions are advisable. If an epileptic has fits at night, it is advisable (but not always possible) that he should sleep under observation. Pillows should be hard to minimize the risk of suffocation.

The amount of freedom the person has depends upon the frequency and timing of his fits, their severity and his behaviour after them. Boxing and football should be forbidden because of blows to the head. The epileptic should not swim or paddle alone. Alcohol should not be taken.

Treatment during a fit

I. MAJOR FIT

If there is time to catch the patient before he falls, he should be placed on the ground. His collar should be loosened. No attempt should be made to control his movements unless he is likely to injure himself; if he is in a place of danger he should be lifted or pulled away. No attempt should be made to force a spoon or wedge between his teeth: if he has bitten his tongue the damage is already done, and trying to force something hard into his mouth can break a tooth. During the clonic stage something soft, such as a folded handkerchief or the corner of a towel, can be slipped between his teeth during a period of muscular relaxation. When the fit is over he should be examined for cuts, bruises, fractures and dislocations. He should remain under observation until he is fully conscious.

2. MINOR FIT

No special treatment is required.

3. STATUS EPILEPTICUS

If the patient is not in hospital he should be moved to one, for it is not possible to say how long an attack will last. A soap-and-water enema can be given: it seems to stop some attacks and does no harm. If fits continue the following drugs can be used:

a. diazepam (Valium) in doses of 10 mg intramuscularly or intravenously, repeatable after 30 minutes;

b. paraldehyde 10 ml intramuscularly; it is slower to act and lasts longer than diazepam; it can cause tissue damage at the site of injection.

Where facilities are available the attack is treated by modern anaesthetic techniques, including giving muscular relaxants and controlled respiration.

Complications are prevented and life maintained by:

provision of adequate airway,	change of posture,
removal of mucus from pharynx,	atropine,
attention to pressure points,	sponging,
antibiotics,	tube-feeding.

Chapter 13 · Presenile dementias

Presenile dementias are certain degenerative diseases of the brain occurring before the age of 65. The most important are:

Alzheimer's disease,
Pick's disease,
Jakob-Creutzfeldt's disease,
Huntington's chorea.

The term presenile covers the period from 45 to 65 years, but presenile dementias, typically both clinically and pathologically, have been described in both younger and older people. All are progressive and incurable.

Other diseases which sometimes resemble presenile dementia are a cerebral tumour, an extradural haematoma, neurosyphilis, cerebral arteriosclerosis, myxoedema, and chronic alcoholism; and tests are carried out to exclude these.

Alzheimer's disease

In this presenile dementia brain cells atrophy and die, and are replaced by fibrous tissue. The neurofibrils in nerve cells are thickened, and plaques of fatty material appear. The brain becomes small, with narrow convolutions and wide sulci. The ventricles of the brain become dilated. Air studies of the brain show the atrophy and ventricular dilatation.

CLINICAL FEATURES

The symptoms and signs are those of dementia. The onset is slow. Typical features are:

loss of memory,
lack of initiative,
carelessness,
antisocial acts, such as petty thefts, exhibitionism, and offences against children,

mood changes,
muscular weaknesses,
tremor,
difficulty in dressing,
fits,
inability to grasp problems,

decline in efficiency,	difficulty in walking,
paranoid ideas,	difficulty in feeding,
speech difficulties,	loss of sphincter control.
rigidity,	

Eventually a profound dementia is produced. Death usually occurs within 5 years of the onset.

TREATMENT

The patient should be looked after at home for as long as possible, and is then admitted to a psychiatric hospital. Treatment is directed towards maintaining nutrition, avoiding injuries, allaying excitement by tranquillizers and sedatives, and preventing bedsores.

Pick's disease

In this disease the atrophy of the brain is more restricted to small areas and is most marked in the frontal and temporal poles.

CLINICAL FEATURES

These are similar to those of Alzheimer's disease, but the patient is likely early on to show fits, incontinence, neurological signs, aphasia, apraxia, and agnosia.

TREATMENT

As for Alzheimer's disease.

Jakob-Creutzfeldt's disease

This disease is less common than Alzheimer's disease and Pick's disease. It is thought to be due to a virus. There is a degeneration and death of cells in many parts of the brain and spinal cord.

CLINICAL FEATURES

The patient shows a progressive dementia and evidence of pyramidal and extrapyramidal disease in the form of motor impairment, speech defect, spasticity, tremor, ataxia, choreo-athetotic movements, and parkinsonism. The combination of a parkinsonian face and profound dementia is typical. Death usually occurs within 9 months.

Huntington's chorea

This is a familial disease transmitted by a dominant gene and therefore inherited by half the children of an affected person. It will occasionally skip a generation or occur spontaneously as the result of a gene change. The brain shows degeneration of the cortex and basal ganglia.

CLINICAL FEATURES

These usually begin at 40–60 years. The disease is characterized by:

> chorea,
> dementia.

Choreic movements can appear before or after the appearance of dementia. They can begin in the face, limbs or trunk, and on one side before the other. Slight early movements are replaced by more violent, abrupt, extensive and disabling movements. Sometimes they are more athetoid than choreic. Voluntary movement is interrupted and disorganized; speech becomes increasingly difficult; gait becomes irregular and erratic.

Dementia shows itself with loss of memory, irresponsibility, apathy, slovenliness, carelessness, hoarding of rubbish. Suicide, self-mutilation, alcoholic sprees, aggressive outbursts and homicidal acts can occur.

Eventually the patient becomes completely helpless, grossly demented, and flung about by violent movements. The deterioration is usually progressive, but it may occasionally appear to be stationary for several years. The duration of the illness is 10–20 years, and death is usually due to an infection.

TREATMENT

This is as for the other dementias. Tranquillizers are given to control the movements. Special care has to be given to the prevention of bedsores, which may be caused by the violent movements chafing the skin.

Chapter 14 · Mental disorders of old age

Old people have many disadvantages. Most of them live on much reduced incomes. Many live in houses that are too big or awkward for them to manage. They are likely to go deaf or have impaired eyesight. They may develop incoordination and attacks of giddiness, and are liable to fall and sustain a fracture. Their hands may tremble. They may be taking an inadequate diet because they have little knowledge of food values, cannot afford good food, have had to give up cooking, or cannot chew because their dentures fit badly. They may be lonely and without relatives or friends, and they may have nothing to do. Failing mental and physical power is likely to cause:

anxiety,   moodiness,
irritability,   insomnia.

The mental disorders they develop are:

senile dementia,   arteriosclerotic dementia,
depressive state,   manic state,
paranoid state,   confusional state.
neurosis,

Senile dementia

This is a dementia beginning usually after the age of 65. The causes are unknown; hereditary factors appear to play a part. More women than men are affected.

The brain shows a generalized cortical atrophy, narrow convolutions and wide sulci. There is little apparent connection between the degree of atrophy and the degree of dementia. The atrophy is due to the degeneration and death of cells in the cortex.

CLINICAL FEATURES

Onset: usually slow.

Course: progressive, can cause profound dementia within a few months.

Intelligence: rapid decline, with narrowing of interests and inability to cope with new problems.

Memory: rapid deterioration, sometimes more for recent events than for old ones, but sometimes 'global', i.e. total.

Emotions: often disturbed. Swings of mood common. Prone to peevishness and irritability. Agitation and depression can occur.

Behaviour: often disturbed. Patient may wander round house, turn on gas taps, shout out of the window, wander about the streets. Restlessness may be due to constipation, faecal obstruction, and (in men) urinary obstruction from an enlarged prostate gland. Repressed tendencies may appear, e.g. stealing, exhibitionism, sexual assaults on children, homosexuality. Apathy common in late stages.

Delusions: commonly of poisoning, maltreatment, theft of personal possessions.

Sleep: insomnia and inverted sleep rhythm.

Speech: vague, irrelevant, confused, and in the end a babble of sound.

Acute confusional state: the patient becomes confused, disorientated, noisy and restless.

Physical health: deteriorates. The patient becomes thin; sphincter control is lost; constipation and faecal impaction can occur; falls cause fractures, especially of the neck of the femur.

Death: Occurs usually within 18 months, due to a pulmonary or other infection, or to inanition and bedsores.

TREATMENT

The patient should be looked after at home or by relatives for as long as conditions and his behaviour allow. Food should contain adequate amounts of protein, milk, fresh vegetables, fruit and vitamins. The bowels should be kept open by giving bran, by laxatives and enemata if necessary. Exercise should be taken in the open air in favourable weather. Accidents should be avoided by removing loose rugs or trailing flex.

Insomnia may be prevented by a small tot of whisky, rum or brandy, or by chloral hydrate 1.0–2.0 g or Mogadon 2.5–5 mg. Restlessness may be reduced by tranquillizers, such as chlorpromazine 25 mg three times a day rising to 50 mg three times a day; overdosing can cause confusion.

When a patient is admitted into hospital, his relatives should be told that admission may precipitate further and rapid deterioration, for about half the patients admitted die within 6 months. The patient should be kept ambulant for as long as possible. Special care has to be given to the prevention of bedsores.

Arteriosclerotic dementia

Arteriosclerotic dementia is due to cerebral arteriosclerosis, either alone or associated with hypertension. Degenerative changes are present in the arteries supplying the brain, which receives an inadequate amount of blood. Areas of softening occur, into which haemorrhages can take place. There may be signs of arteriosclerosis in other parts of the body.

CLINICAL FEATURES

Clinically arteriosclerotic dementia is distinguished from senile dementia in several ways: it is always associated with arteriosclerosis, affects men more often than women, begins at an earlier age, is episodic rather than continuous in its manifestations, and does not affect the personality of the patient until it is well advanced.

Course: is intermittent, with deterioration following each exacerbation.

Intelligence: declines; loss of interests, inability to grasp new ideas.

Memory: declines, especially for recent events.

Insight: is occasionally present in the early stages, and likely to cause anxiety and depression.

Behaviour: deterioration in personal care, slovenliness, over-reaction to alcohol, exhibitionsim, homosexual behaviour, sexual assaults on children.

Mood: can be depression or inappropriate elation.

Acute confusional state: an attack of confusion, disorientation, restlessness, delusions and hallucinations, lasting for days or weeks.

Local lesions of brain: liable to produce hemiplegia, facial paralysis, spasticity, parkinsonism, tremors, fits.

Hypertension: liable to produce headaches, unsteadiness, giddiness and blackouts. Attacks of *hypertensive encephalopathy* can occur, with a steep rise in BP, vomiting, headache, blindness, fits and paralysis; last for some hours; are likely to produce permanent paralysis.

Death: from pneumonia, renal failure, cardiac failure or cerebral haemorrhage.

TREATMENT

The treatment is predominantly medical, with appropriate drugs for hypertension and a readjustment of the patient's life to his disability. The patient's work and responsibilities should be diminished or given up. Rest in bed is necessary in the acute phases. The patient should be looked after at home for as long as possible.

Depressive and manic states

Depressive and manic states occur in old age as in younger people. They can be first attacks or repetitions of previous attacks.

Attacks of depression are more common than attacks of mania. They can be precipitated by retirement, bereavement, illness, operations, poverty and loneliness. They may be typical depressions of the manic-depressive psychosis variety, with depressive ideas and retardation, or they may present as an agitated, anxious depression with paranoid ideas and delusions of bizarre physical disease. When the presenting symptoms are anxiety, insomnia, and a preoccupation with physical functions, the condition may be thought to be an anxiety state. Suicide is common in depressive illnesses in old age.

Mania is similar to that of earlier years, with a sudden onset, flight of ideas, delusions of wealth and power, sometimes amorous advances, and often a sudden termination. An attack sometimes becomes chronic.

Treatment follows the usual lines for depressive and manic illnesses. Old age is not *per se* a bar to ECT, a few treatments often producing a rapid improvement.

Paranoid states

A paranoid state can develop for the first time in an old person. It is more common in women than men. The condition can be regarded as a schizophrenic illness. Isolation by blindness or deafness can be a factor.

The patient becomes solitary and suspicious, and then goes on to develop delusions of persecution, as a result of which he becomes solitary, detached, and sometimes abusive or threatening, and he may barricade himself into his room or house. He is completely without insight; but he may retain his personality and habits in all matters unconnected with his delusional ideas.

Admission to hospital is usually necessary. The prognosis is bad. Recovery is rare.

Confusional states

Acute confusional states are common in old age. They can be caused by organic diseases of the brain, acute infections, heart failure, a fracture, a major surgical operation, gross vitamin deficiency, and over-sensitivity to or over-dosage by drugs. Drugs that can cause a confusional state include:

tranquillizers,	antidepressants,
antidiabetic drugs,	antiparkinsonian drugs,
cortisone,	diphenylhydantoin
barbiturates,	bromides.

CLINICAL FEATURES

The onset of an attack is usually spread over a few days. Early symptoms are irritability, restlessness, insomnia and loss of appetite. At the height of the attack the patient is incoherent, grossly confused, disorientated and hallucinated. He takes little or no food, can become severely dehydrated, and develops rectal impaction of faeces. The death rate is high, but with treatment, recovery is possible. An incurable dementia can follow an attack.

TREATMENT

The patient is admitted into hospital, and given adequate fluids and food, with additional vitamin intake. Any drug which may have caused the attack is stopped, unless a sudden discontinuation, e.g. of insulin or a steroid, would be dangerous. Constipation is relieved by enema; impacted faeces are removed. Sedation is usually by paraldehyde 2–8 ml because it is a relatively safe drug.

Neuroses in old age

The patient may have shown neurotic reactions in earlier life. If he develops a neurosis in old age for the first time, it is likely that his symptoms are really those of a depression or of a physical illness. Anxiety states and obsessional-compulsive states are the usual neurotic illnesses of old age; hysteria is seen less commonly.

TREATMENT

Treatment of a neurosis in old age is as much a social as a medical problem. Social provisions for old people—such as home helps, clubs and recreational facilities—do much to prevent the formation of neurotic patterns or to relieve them when they have occurred. Individual psychotherapy of a simple kind may be given. The patient's physical health should be maintained at as high a level as possible.

Chapter 15 · Other organic diseases

Mental symptoms occur in a number of physical diseases with such intensity that they form a prominent part of the illness or by occurring before physical signs appear cause a physical illness to be mistaken for a psychiatric one. A physical examination of the patient is essential on admission to hospital, and when the doctor is in any doubt about the diagnosis it should be repeated in as detailed a form as necessary or the patient's condition allows; appropriate special investigations are carried out.

Infective-exhaustive psychosis

An infective-exhaustive psychosis can occur in acute infections, especially of the nervous system (encephalitis, meningitis, brain abscess), and in extreme physical exhaustion.

CLINICAL FEATURES

The patient looks physically ill, with a rapid pulse, sweating and tremor of hands and lips; in infections the temperature is raised. Likely psychiatric symptoms are:

confusion,	disorientation,
incoherent speech,	irrelevant replies to questions,
emotional lability,	delusions of persecution,
hallucinations,	restlessness,
violence,	coma in severe cases.

When the condition is due to physical exhaustion, likely symptoms are:

irritability,	restlessness,
acute anxiety,	oversensitivity to light and noise.
nightmares,	

TREATMENT

The patient should be nursed in a single room, without bright lights or dark shadows. He will require tranquillizers and sedatives. A prolonged bath is helpful in calming an excited patient and promoting sleep. An enema may be required for constipation, and catheterization is sometimes necessary. Adequate amounts of fluid should be given by mouth, through a tube or by intravenous injection. When the physical state has improved, ECT often clears up any residual psychotic symptoms.

Renal failure

Renal failure (uraemia) is produced by failure of the excretory functions of the kidneys, which can occur in any severe renal disease or when renal function is impaired in shock, heart failure, dehydration, extensive tissue necrosis, etc. Severe biochemical disturbance of the body is produced.

CLINICAL FEATURES

In slowly developing renal failure, early symptoms are fatigue, depression and loss of appetite. When the failure becomes severe the following can occur:

a. nausea, hiccoughing, vomiting, diarrhoea;
b. muscular weakness, twitchings, cramps;
c. heart failure, hypertension, hypertensive encephalopathy, retinitis, oedema, pericarditis;
d. anaemia, purpura, bleeding from nose, gums and bowel;
e. confusion, fits, coma.

TREATMENT

Treatment is aimed at eliminating toxic substances from the body and at maintaining electrolyte and water balance. The methods used are (a) peritoneal dialysis, in which fluid is run in and out of the peritoneal cavity, (b) an artificial kidney machine, and (c) transplantation of a kidney from a suitable donor.

Hepatic failure

Failure of liver function occurs in any severe disease of the liver, the commonest of which is cirrhosis of the liver. Psychiatric features include:

fatigue,	depression,
excitement,	abnormal behaviour,
confusion,	drowsiness.
coma,	

Hepatic coma is often fatal, and if the patient does recover he is likely to suffer another attack.

TREATMENT

Treatment is by the maintenance of fluid and electrolyte balance, the maintenance of carbohydrate intake, and the replacement of any blood lost, in the hope that in the meantime the liver cells will grow again and liver function be restored.

Anoxia

Anoxia (lack of oxygen) occurs in carbon monoxide poisoning and by reaching a high altitude in mountaineering or flying without additional sources of oxygen.

CLINICAL FEATURES

These can be early or late.
Early features: impairment of judgment and perception, loss of efficiency, loss of self-control, lethargy, confusion, loss of consciousness, vomiting, coma.
Late features: these can occur weeks or months later and are due to degeneration of brain cells. Symptoms are headache, giddiness, confusion, disorientation, parkinsonian syndrome with rigidity of muscles, immobile features, speech disturbance and dementia. The condition is irreversible and permanent.

TREATMENT

The patient is removed from the cause of the anoxia and given oxygen.

Hyperthyroidism

Hyperthyroidism is the condition produced by excessive amounts of thyroid hormones in the blood. The cause is unknown. It can be familial. Its onset is sometimes associated with mental stress or trauma, but the association may be a coincidence. Psychiatric features resemble an acute anxiety state.

CLINICAL FEATURES

These are physical and mental.
Physical features are:

enlargement of the thyroid gland in most cases,
prominence of the eyes,
rapid, irregular heart rate,
itching,
tremor,
sweating,
menorrhagia or amenorrhoea.

Mental symptoms are:

fatigue,
anxiety,
hypomanic moods,
delirium,
irritability,
insomnia, disturbed sleep,
hysterical reactions.

TREATMENT

Treatment is by (a) antithyroid drugs (e.g. methyl thiouracil) for 1–2 years, (b) radioactive iodine to destroy thyroid cells, or (c) subtotal thyroidectomy, about 95 per cent of the gland being removed. Thyroidectomy may relieve psychotic features, but sometimes precipitates them.

Myxoedema

Myxoedema is hypothyroidism in adults and is due to a failure of the thyroid gland to produce an adequate amount of its hormones.

CLINICAL FEATURES

The course is slow and insidious, except when the disease is due to thyroidectomy, treatment by radioiodine, or a thyroiditis. Features are physical and mental.
Physical features are:

constipation,	obesity,
aching pains,	loss of hair,
thick lips,	coarse features,
croaking voice,	snoring,
dry skin,	swollen joints.
sensitivity to cold,	

Mental features are:

intellectual decline,
loss of memory,
'myxoedemic madness'—delusions of persecution, hallucinations, confusion and violence,
apathy,
inactivity.

TREATMENT

Thyroxine sodium 15–300 μg is given daily by mouth. Improvement should be noticed within a few weeks. Maintenance doses are given for life.

Cushing's syndrome

In this syndrome there is an over-production of cortisone by the adrenal glands, either from an adrenal tumour or by over-stimulation by the pituitary gland.

CLINICAL FEATURE

Features are physical and mental.
Physical features are:

obesity of face, neck, trunk,	bruising,
decalcification of bone,	amenorrhoea,

purple striae in skin,   acne,
diabetes mellitus,   virilization in women.

Mental features include:

fatigue,   apathy.
depression (sometimes to
    suicidal intensity),

TREATMENT

An adrenal gland tumour is removed. Irradiation of the pituitary gland is performed when the gland is the cause of the disease.

Pernicious anaemia

Patients with pernicious anaemia can show depression, irritability, manic state, paranoid state or mild delirium. Mental features can occur long before other evidence of the disease is obvious. Symptoms should clear up rapidly when vitamin B_{12} is given.

Cerebral tumour

Psychiatric symptoms are sometimes the first and occasionally the only symptoms of a cerebral tumour. They may precede by weeks or months any neurological findings, and it is not unusual for a diagnosis of a psychosis or neurosis to be made. The particular symptoms produced will be decided by the nature of the tumour, the speed of its growth, and its position in the brain and into which it may spread. Psychiatric symptoms are especially likely if the tumour arises in the frontal lobe, the corpus callosum and the temporo-parietal region. They are less likely when it originates in the occipital lobe and the cerebellum.
Mental features are:

tumour in frontal lobe and corpus callosum

loss of memory,   anxiety,
personality changes,   euphoria,
childishness,   tactlessness,
irritability,   excitement.

temporal lobe tumours

> temporal lobe epilepsy,   speech disturbances if domi-
> nant lobe is affected.

Physical features are:

headache,	nausea, vomiting,
fits,	papilloedema,
paralyses,	excessive sleep.

TREATMENT

Surgical removal of affected part of brain is performed if possible.

Multiple sclerosis

Multiple (disseminated) sclerosis is a common disease of the nervous system. Its cause is unknown. The first attack usually occurs at 15–30 years. Subsequent attacks can occur at any time. An attack commonly clears up in a few weeks, and may leave little or no trace. Most patients are only slightly affected, but a few become severely crippled. During an attack areas of the brain become inflamed, and when the inflammation settles down the affected part may become sclerosed (hardened) by the development of fibrous tissue.

CLINICAL FEATURES

These are varied and can be slight or severe.
Common physical features are:

slight visual disturbance,	frequency and urgency
numbness or weakness of limb,	of micturition,
giddiness,	tremor,
	spastic paralysis.

Common mental features are:

emotional disturbances,	euphoria,
apathy,	irritability,
difficulty in concentrating,	depression.
intellectual deterioration,	

An acute attack can present the picture of an infective-exhaustive psychosis.

TREATMENT

No known treatment affects the course of the disease. During an attack rest in bed is advisable. Between attacks avoidance of physical exertion, rest periods and warm baths are advised. A severely crippled patient requires full nursing care.

Paralysis agitans

Paralysis agitans (Parkinson's disease) is a progressive disease of the brain due to degeneration in the basal ganglia and cortex. The cause is unknown. There is thought to be a chemical imbalance in some brain cells. The usual age of onset is 45–65 years. It occurs in about 1 per cent of people over 50. In some people it is due to athero-sclerosis of cerebral arteries, haemorrhage into the ganglia, and carbon monoxide poisoning. *Parkinsonism*, in a mild and usually reversible form, can be caused by some tranquillizers and antidepressants.

CLINICAL FEATURES

The onset is slow and is not usually noticed by the patient. When fully developed the condition is easy to recognize.

PHYSICAL FEATURES

The principal features are tremor and rigidity.
Tremor: fine or moderate in degree; present at rest, disappears on voluntary movement; limited for a time to one limb or side; eventually involves the whole body.
Rigidity: muscular movements performed slowly; speaking, chewing and swallowing are hampered; speech becomes monotonous; patient's face becomes masklike, with unblinking eyes and ordinary lines washed out.
Posture: trunk is held in a stoop.
Walking: little, shuffling steps.
Mental features: the patient is liable to become depressed, peevish and sometimes suicidal. In prolonged cases, dementia appears.

TREATMENT

Light massage, passive movements and warm baths are helpful. Anti-parkinsonian drugs are used and affect the rigidity more than the tremor. They include:

> levodopa: 0.25 g twice daily, increasing to 2.5–5.0 g daily in divided doses,
> amantadine hydrochloride (Symmetrel): 200–600 mg daily,
> benzhexol hydrochloride (Artane, Pipanol) 2–15 mg daily in divided doses,
> orphenadrine hydrochloride (Disipal): 100–300 mg daily in divided doses.

Several drugs may have to be tried before an effective one is found.

Dystrophia myotonica

This is a form of muscular dystrophy. It is familial and usually appears at 20–30 years. Patients show muscular wasting, myotonia (an inability to relax contracted muscles), premature baldness, testicular atrophy, and cataracts. They are very likely to become paranoid. There is no treatment.

Systemic lupus erythematosus

Systemic lupus erythematosus (SLE) is a collagen disease most common in women aged 20–50. It can run a benign course for years, with sometimes stationary periods, but in some cases it runs a rapid and progressive course, causing death within two years.

CLINICAL FEATURES

A rash appears on the face; it is reddish, hard and raised and has a 'butterfly' distribution on the nose and cheeks. In acute phases the patient is ill with fever and enlarged joints. Other evidence of disease can appear in the kidneys, lungs, heart, liver, blood and nervous system.

Mental features: anxiety, depression, confusion and delusions can occur.

TREATMENT

Treatment is by bed rest, analgesics for arthritis and pain. Cortisones and chloroquine are given.

Bromide poisoning

Bromides are not now medically prescribed, but they may be ingredients of 'nerve tonics', and self-administration can be a cause of poisoning. They are particularly dangerous for old people, for arteriosclerotics, and for people with renal disease.

CLINICAL FEATURES

The following can occur:

headache,	restlessness,
irritability,	euphoria,
slurred speech,	insomnia,
confusion,	disorientation,
delirium,	hallucinations.

The diagnosis is confirmed by examining the level of bromide in the blood. The normal blood bromide is below 50 mg per ml. One of 100 mg is suspect, and one of 200 mg and over is definitely toxic.

TREATMENT

The drug is stopped immediately. Sodium chloride is given by mouth and fluids pushed.

Lead poisoning

Lead poisoning can be due to absorption from industrial processes, to licking lead-containing paint, and to contamination of food and drink by lead-glazed pots and lead pipes.

CLINICAL FEATURES

These include anaemia, malnutrition, muscular pains, abdominal colic, and constipation. Acute lead poisoning produces an acute encephalopathy with hemiplegia, cranial nerve paralyses, fits, blindness, coma and death. Lead poisoning in infancy and early childhood is thought to be a possible cause of mental handicap.

TREATMENT

This is by removal from the source of lead, treatment with a chelating agent (which promotes the excretion of lead), and relief of colic and muscular pain.

Mental disorders of menstruation and childbearing

CHILDBEARING

In spite of the emotional problems it can arouse, this is not often a cause of mental illness. During pregnancy many women feel particularly well and some neurotics are improved while they are pregnant. A psychosis may develop before or after childbirth. It may be a mild toxic-confusional state, a depression, a mania or schizophrenia. The psychosis is usually mild with a good prognosis. But a depression may be acute and the woman may kill her child and commit suicide.

PREMENSTRUAL TENSION

This is a common condition. It occurs regularly in some women, who for a few days before the onset of menstruation are tense, anxious, irritable and discontented. The symptoms disappear with the onset of menstruation. It is thought to be due to hormonal imbalance during the second half of the menstrual cycle. Some women show a lack of progesterone during the period, but in others the progesterone level is normal. Some patients are relieved by the administration of progesterone. Another method is by taking the combined oestrogen-progestogen birth control pill, thus avoiding ovulation and menstruation.

Psychiatric disorders in surgery and intensive care

Psychiatric disorders can complicate:

transplant surgery,   chest surgery,

| coronary thrombosis, | hysterectomy, |
| renal dialysis, | removal of cataract. |

Anxiety, depression, confusion and delirium can occur. The staff of intensive care and other specialized units can develop psychiatric symptoms. Intensive care is very responsible work and places great stress on the nursing staff. Patients are inevitably very ill and require constant and careful attention. The nurse must always be alert and watchful, and ready to take swift action in a crisis. In addition she must be able to handle sophisticated equipment competently. Dealing with distressed and anxious relatives, trying to reassure them and give them sympathy and understanding in an already stressful situation, makes great demands on the nurse, and it is not surprising that the mental and emotional strain should take its toll.

Chapter 16 · Mental handicap

Mental handicap is also called mental retardation, mental deficiency and subnormality.

The mentally handicapped are those people whose intelligence does not develop to the normal level. The IQ (intelligence quotient) is an approximate measure of a person's intelligence. If we take the average person to have an IQ in the 75–125 range, the mentally handicapped have an IQ below 75. There are two dissimilar and distinct groups:

> high grade people with IQ 75–50,
> medium and low grade people with IQ below 50.

Incidence

About 5 per cent of all babies born have a congenital disability of mind or body. Many of these have severe physical abnormalities (such as deformities of the heart) and die in infancy or childhood, their deaths reducing the number of handicapped children to 1–4 per cent. Adult mentally handicapped people form about 1 per cent of all adults.

HIGH GRADE PEOPLE

These are more likely to be educational and social problems than nursing and medical ones. Essentially they are normal people at the dull end, and they are no more abnormal than the clever people at the bright end. They are usually the children of dull parents, their condition being genetically determined.

Physical appearance
They are usually physically normal. The less intelligent may be below average height and may show an increased incidence of epilepsy.

Mental development
In infancy they appear to be normal, but they are slower than

average people in the rate of development and in the acquisition of skills such as speaking and walking. Their disability may be unnoticed if their parents and siblings (brothers and sisters) are dull, but it will show if the rest of the family are intelligent. They do poorly at school and may require special education. On leaving school they may have difficulty in finding employment. Stable adults settle in some job which does not require much intelligence and may happily work at it for life. They tend to marry their own kind and to have the same kind of children. Should such a person come into hospital, it is well to consider that he may not be able to read fluently, to follow complicated directions, to be able to give himself injections of insulin, and may become bewildered by the hospital environment.

If these patients are unstable they can present problems. They may have left home or been thrown out by their parents. They tend to change jobs frequently, throwing them up for trivial reasons or being dismissed for incompetence and rudeness. They may break down into acute emotional outbursts. Some become aggressive psychopaths.

MEDIUM AND LOW GRADE PATIENTS

The IQ of medium grade patients is 50–25. The IQ of low grade patients is below 25.

Medium grade patients can look after themselves in simple ways. They can learn to wash, dress and feed themselves. The brightest of them will learn to speak simple sentences, to print their names, to recognize some words and coins. They can be taught to do simple work, and often excel at repetitive tasks.

Low grade patients are completely dependent upon others. Many of them have to be fed, washed, cleansed and dressed. Incontinence of urine and faeces is common. They cannot be taught to read and write. Some are quiet and friendly. Others are noisy, excitable, vicious and destructive; they may swallow rubbish.

The lower the patient's intelligence the more likely he is to show physical deformities.

Height: below average.

Facies: mis-shapen; head abnormally small or large or irregular; eyes abnormally shaped; ears abnormally shaped or positioned; hair coarse.

Mouth: teeth erupt late and badly placed; high incidence of caries; palate high and narrow.

Epilepsy: common.
Spasticity: common.
Skin: coarse and thick.
Heart: high incidence of congenital abnormalities.

Causes of mental handicap

1. GENETIC FACTORS

Genes are transmitted to the infant in the chromosomes of the sex cells of its parents. Genes are liable to mutation (change), and some of these mutations cause mental handicap. Genes may be dominant: when a person has a dominant gene it is transmitted to half his or her children, who will be affected by it and will be liable to pass it on to half their children; the other children will not be affected by it and will not pass it on. Genes may be recessive: a recessive gene does not cause any ill effect unless the child receives it from both parents, and the chance of this happening in parents unrelated by blood is remote. When both parents have the same recessive gene, about 1 child in 4 is likely to be affected. A gene can mutate spontaneously, without the abnormality being inherited, and a disease can then appear in a family in which it has not appeared before.

2. CONDITIONS OCCURRING DURING FETAL LIFE

Certain conditions occurring during fetal life can produce mental handicap in the child. These include German measles, cytomegalovirus infection, toxoplasmosis, syphilis, kernicterus, maternal alcoholism, and X-rays of abdomen and pelvis.

The fetus is particularly vulnerable during the first 3 months of its life, while its tissues and organs are developing into their normal patterns and functions.

3. CONDITIONS OCCURRING AT BIRTH

A baby's brain may be damaged during birth, especially if the birth is premature, precipitate or prolonged, if forceps have to be used, or if the baby is born as a breech presentation. The cells of the baby's brain can be affected by anoxia (lack of oxygen) and by haemorrhages into and around it.

4. CONDITIONS OCCURRING AFTER BIRTH

These can be meningitis, encephalitis, injuries to the brain and lead poisoning. In these children there can be a history of normal development up to the onset of the precipitating illness. After the onset of the illness the child may develop more slowly than he should or cease to develop any more or regress to a lower mental level.

Special types of mental handicap

Down's syndrome (mongolism, trisomy-21 syndrome)

Down's syndrome occurs in about 1 in every 600 babies born. The patient has an extra chromosome of the 21 group. In some cases the extra chromosome is attached to another chromosome, the state being called translocation. When the extra chromosome is not translocated, there is an association with the age of the mother, for the incidence of the condition rises sharply after the maternal age of 35, and at 40 the incidence is 1 in 60 births. When the extra chromosome is translocated, the condition may be inherited from either the mother or the father. Sometimes not all cells show the extra chromosome, and this is called mosaicism.

Patients with Down's syndrome look very much like one another, although every one does not show all the features of the condition. Typical are short stature; round head, broad nose, sparse hair; eyes sloping downwards and inwards, an epicanthic fold of skin at the inner corner of the eye, nystagmus, squint, small cataracts; tongue fissured and too large for the mouth; hands broad and short, single crease across the palm, short incurved little finger; short neck and trunk; hypotonic muscles; poor peripheral circulation.

Congenital disease of heart and bowel is common. Leukaemia can occur.

Almost all patients with Down's syndrome are moderately or severely mentally handicapped. As babies they are placid, apathetic and inactive. In personality they do not differ from other mentally handicapped people.

Prevention is by the identification of parents at risk—those in whose families Down's syndrome has occurred and when the mother is over the age of 35. A specimen of amniotic fluid is examined for chromosomes in cells from the fetal skin. If the additional chromosome is found, indicating the fetus has Down's syndrome, an abortion could be offered to the parents. If women stopped having babies over the age of 35, there would be a marked fall in the number of affected babies born.

Klinefelter's syndrome

This condition occurs in men only. They have two X chromosomes instead of one, as well as the Y chromosome. Most of them are mentally normal; a few have some degree of mental handicap. They are thin, with poor sexual development, small testes, infertility and female breast development. A married one may present himself at an infertility clinic because his wife does not become pregnant.

Turner's syndrome

This affects women only. An affected woman has one X chromosome instead of two. She shows dwarfism, underdeveloped ovaries, and webbing of the neck. She may be of normal intelligence.

Triple X syndrome (super-female syndrome)

Affected women have three X chromosomes instead of two. They are of normal physical appearance. Some are mentally handicapped. They can have normal children.

Cerebral palsy

A patient with cerebral palsy shows spastic paralysis, often associated with involuntary athetoid or choreic movements. About three-quarters of them are mentally handicapped in degrees varying from slight to severe.

Many cases are genetically determined. A few are due to anoxia of the brain during childbirth, to encephalitis, meningitis and brain injury. The brain is likely to show developmental errors such as small gyri, areas of softening or hardening, cysts and hydro-cephaly.

The patient develops spastic paralyis due to damage to motor neurones or their failure to develop. According to the parts involved, the following names are given:

diplegia: both arms or both legs affected;
monoplegia: one limb only affected;
hemiplegia: arm and leg on the same side affected;
triplegia: three limbs affected;
quadriplegia: all limbs affected.

When the condition is congenital, it is recognizable within a few months of birth. The child walks late. Walking on the toes is common. The thighs may be adducted, the child walking with a 'scissors gait' of crossed thighs. The paralysed limbs are held rigid by muscles that are continually in spasm; sleep does not bring any relaxation. The patient can have difficulty in speaking, chewing, swallowing, and walking.

Involuntary movements are common. They can be athetoid (slow, twisting, writhing), choreic (short, jerky), or both. They severely hinder any voluntary movement. They become worse if the patient becomes emotionally upset.

Epilepsy is common.

Psychological assessment is difficult, and commonly the patient appears to be less intelligent than he is.

Kernicterus

This is a condition produced by brain damage caused by severe jaundice in the newly-born. The jaundice is due to Rhesus incom-patibility, to giving excessive amounts of vitamin K to a mother in labour or to a newly born baby, and to dehydration and sepsis in the newly born. Damage is done to areas of grey matter within the cerebral hemispheres.

Untreated infants show evidence within the first few weeks of life. Untreated they develop deep jaundice, have a temperature, twitch, arch the back or have fits; many die. Survivors are likely to have mental handicap, athetoid or choreic movements, spastic paralysis and epilepsy.

PREVENTION

Rhesus incompatibility is produced when a Rh negative woman becomes pregnant by a Rh positive man and the fetus inherits a Rh positive factor from the father. The first child is unaffected, but at the time of the separation of the placenta at its birth enough fetal blood gets into the mother's circulation to produce substances called antibodies. Subsequent babies are at risk, for these antibodies can pass into the fetal circulation, destroy the baby's red blood cells and so cause jaundice.

The Rh factor of a pregnant woman is determined. If it is negative, the Rh factor of the father is determined. If his is positive, the woman is at risk in further pregnancies if she is not treated after the birth of the child. Within 36 hours of the birth she is injected with human gammaglobulin containing anti-D antibodies. This destroys the fetal cells in her blood and prevents her from developing the harmful antibodies.

If this has not been done and a baby develops severe jaundice, it is necessary to do an 'exchange transfusion', the baby's blood being replaced via the umbilical vein with an equal amount of Rh negative blood.

German measles (rubella) syndrome

If a pregnant woman develops German measles during the first 3 months of pregnancy, serious damage can be done to the child. After 3 months any damage is likely to be slight. About 1 child in 10 at risk shows abnormalities, which can be severe mental handicap, low birth weight, microcephaly, small eyes, cataracts, deafness, deaf-mutism, harelip, cleft palate, congenital heart disease.

Prevention is by the vaccination of all girls with the German measles virus before they reach child-bearing age.

Cytomegalovirus infection

This virus is widely distributed. Infection of an adult causes little or no apparent illness. About 1 per cent of pregnant women become infected during pregnancy, and about half their children become affected before birth. Of these infected children 5–15 per cent are brain-damaged. The virus is responsible for 200–600 mentally handicapped children in Britain every year. Abnormalities produced are: mental handicap of varying degree, microcephaly, low birth-weight, meningo-encephalitis, spasticity, epilepsy.

There is no way of preventing the infection.

Toxoplasmosis

This is due to infection by a protozoon called *Toxoplasma gondii*. Infection of man is thought to be from cats. It can produce mental handicap, microcephaly or hydrocephaly, and epilepsy. The brain shows inflammatory lesions, which in time become calcified and are then visible on X-ray.

Congenital syphilis

This is now rare where there are good facilities for the investigation and treatment of syphilis. Affected children who survive birth and early infancy are likely to show mental handicap, poor sight and hearing, and deformities of bone. Further mental decline can set in in infancy.

Prevention: a Wassermann Reaction (WR) or other test for syphilis is carried out on pregnant women and if it is found to be positive, the woman is given antisyphilitic treatment. *Treatment* of an affected baby is by penicillin or other appropriate antibiotic.

Phenylketonuria

This is a metabolic disease due to the absence of an enzyme which converts phenylalanine, and amino acid present in many foods, into tyrosine. In consequence phenylalanine accumulates and damages the brain. Untreated patients are likely to show:

> mental handicap: severe, with many mannerisms,
> fair skin and light hair,
> eczema,
> microcephaly.

About 97 per cent of patients answer to the above description, and respond to treatment. About 3 per cent have different enzymal deficiencies and suffer from a malignant phenylketonuria with progressive neurological degeneration, hypotonia and fits; the decline is not affected by adequate dietary control, and almost all die before they are 7. Some people have been found (by chemical tests) to have a slight or transient phenylketonuria and did not show deterioration although they were not treated.

Chemically the diagnosis is made by the Guthrie test on the baby's blood, by estimation of the blood phenylalanine level, and by special tests to disclose if the condition is or is not malignant.

Treatment is by putting the affected baby on a phenylalanine-free diet and keeping him on it for several years. The complete exclusion of phenylalanine is not advisable for when it is tried the baby does not thrive, has feeding difficulties, and can develop eczema.

Cretinism

Cretinism is produced by inadequate secretion of thyroid hormones in infancy. It is now rare in Britain. Affected children show signs after the age of 3 months. They become dull and apathetic, do not develop mentally at the normal rate, have a stunted growth, low temperature, constipation, coarse features and a croaking voice.

Treatment is by sodium thyroxine by mouth, continued for life.

Hydrocephaly

In this condition there is an excessive amount of cerebrospinal fluid in the brain. It is usually due to a congenital obstruction to the escape of CSF from the ventricles into the subarachnoid space. As a result the CSF accumulates in larger and larger amounts, compressing brain tissue and dilating the ventricles. In some cases it is associated with *spina bifida*, a failure of closure of nervous and skeletal tissue in the lumbar region.

Features of the untreated case are:

enlarging head,	dilated veins on scalp,
non-closure of sutures,	spasticity,
wasting,	epilepsy.
blindness,	

In many cases the enlargement stops spontaneously. In a few

there can be a rapid increase in the size of the head with general physical decline.

Treatment: no specific treatment is advisable if the enlargement is slow or has stopped. In others it is necessary to insert a tube into a ventricle and drain the fluid into a vein.

Microcephaly

Microcephaly means small-headed and many mentally handicapped people have small heads. *True microcephaly* is a condition in which the patient has a characteristic appearance with a long skull, flattened from side to side, prominent nose and upper jaw, and sometimes a receding jaw. The circumference of the head does not exceed 43 cm. The patient is severely mentally handicapped. Epilepsy and spasticity are common complications.

Tuberous sclerosis (epiloia)

This condition is usually due to a new mutation in the sex cells of one or other parent, but it can be inherited as a dominant. Typical features are:

> adenoma sebaceum: pink nodules appearing on the cheeks at 4–5 years, gradually spreading and becoming larger and darker,
> small white patches in the skin, present at birth,
> shagreen patch, of irregularly thickened skin in lumbar region,
> areas of fibrous and later calcified tissue in brain,
> epilepsy,
> intelligence: average in about one-third, declining to severely handicapped.

Intellectually normal members of the family may show some of the skin or other signs of the disease.

Lead Poisoning

Mental handicap can be due to licking or eating paint containing lead; lead in petrol is a possible cause; in some areas the amount of lead in soft water is higher than it should be. Other signs of lead poisoning are ill-health, abdominal pains, confusion and fits.

Alcoholism

Mothers who drink heavily during pregnancy are liable to have children who are mentally handicapped and have microcephaly and congenital abnormalities of the heart and joints.

Brain injury

The brain of a child may be injured by stresses at birth, anoxia at birth, car accidents, baby battering, meningitis and encephalitis. Such injuries can cause mental handicap, spastic paralysis, choreic or athetoid movements, epilepsy and speech difficulties.

The treatment of mental handicap

There are only a few kinds of mental handicap for which it is possible to give specific treatment, e.g. cretinism, phenyl-ketonuria. The care of the handicapped is as much a social and educational matter as a medical and nursing one.

A mentally handicapped person should be looked after at home and in the community if facilities are adequate and the person does not present insuperable problems. The local authority of the area in which he lives should provide many facilities, such as schooling, day hospitals, and hostels and training centres for older people. Parents are likely to need psychological assistance in their emotional difficulties, and material assistance such as better housing, laundry facilities, and the support and advice of health visitor, community nurse and social worker.

Mentally handicapped children and adults can be admitted to a hospital for the mentally handicapped if facilities in the home and community are inadequate, if the parents are incapable of looking after him, if he requires nursing care or special training (such as by behaviour modification), or if his behaviour is such that he cannot stay at home or in a hostel. In the hospital he will receive adequate nursing and medical care, and according to his age, mental state and physical health attend school, training centre, etc. The hospital will have facilities for recreation, sport and work, and aims at providing as full a life as possible for its residents.

Chapter 17 · The psychiatry of childhood

The psychiatric problems presented by children differ from those presented by adults. The child is developing and maturing; he is much influenced by others—by his parents, siblings (brothers and sisters), other relatives, friends, teachers; he is affected by the environment in which he lives.

From his parents a child should expect love, consistent handling and a stable environment. If he does not get them he is likely to be upset. His mother is the most important person in his life. The father is usually less important for he is likely to see him less and to come into a less close personal relationship. The child is likely to be seriously upset if he appreciates that his mother does not love him, that she rejects him, that she wishes he had been of the opposite sex. He can become disturbed if he is inconsistently handled, being at one time loved and accepted and at another rejected. Some parents expect their child always to behave like a little lady or gentleman and to conform to the patterns of behaviour of a much older person, with the result that the child either conforms closely to the expected pattern or reacts violently against it. Other parents are overprotective, not allowing the child to develop independence and still doing for him what he should be capable of learning to do himself. As he grows older and goes to school he is exposed to conflicting patterns and may be expected to behave in different ways at home and at school.

A child may have to live in a socially bad environment or to live with dull, inadequate or abnormal parents. A child's parents may die, be imprisoned or abandon him, and he may be given to the care of others or have to live in an institution. Some children are handicapped by physical diseases such as cerebral palsy, epilepsy, congenital heart disease, diabetes and muscular dystrophy.

The birth of another child to the family can cause the elder child to regress to an earlier stage of development, to baby-talk, or bed-wetting in one who had previously been dry. Any child can react to stress or an emotional problem by exhibiting a disorder of behaviour. Such a reaction can be considered normal. It should be considered to be abnormal if it persists for a long time, if it is very severe, if it occurs long after the age at which it might be expected to occur, or if several reactions occur together. Many a child's emotional reactions are short-lived and disappear as he becomes older or as circumstances improve.

A young child is not likely to present his troubles in words. He usually presents them in his behaviour, and it is usually a disorder of behaviour that gives rise to a suspicion that something is wrong with him. An infant is limited in the ways he can express himself as being unhappy: he can cry, refuse food, vomit, sleep badly, fail to thrive.

Conduct disorders

THUMB SUCKING AND NAIL BITING

Thumb sucking is normal in infancy and a child may suck his thumb in sleep, long after he has given it up when awake. It can persist in an unhappy or tired child. Nail biting is common and occasionally persists into adult life. Like thumb sucking it occurs in unhappy and tired children.

TEMPER TANTRUMS

Temper tantrums occur as normal phenomena in young children from 2 to 5 years. They are precipitated by the child's discovery that his wishes are not immediately gratified: the child has an acute emotional reaction in which he screams, throws himself on the floor, kicks, waves his arms and bangs his head. Such a reaction can disturb a parent who does not expect it or appreciate that at this age it is normal. They can be relieved by the parent building up a secure, loving relationship with the child.

BED-WETTING

Bed-wetting (nocturnal enuresis) is common. A child is usually dry at night at the age of 3, although he may occasionally wet his bed during the next couple of years. About 10 per cent of children wet the bed at 5 years, about 5 per cent at 10 years, and 1–2 per cent in their teens, More than one member of the family may be bed-wetters. Wetting by day (diurnal enuresis) is much less common.

Causes
1. A developmental factor with delayed muscle nerve control of bladder: the majority of cases.
2. Lack of training or faulty training by dull or abnormal parents in bad domestic circumstances.
3. Emotional disturbance—separation from mother, admission into hospital, birth of sibling.
4. Physical disease: physical abnormality of neck of bladder or urethra, urinary infection, epilepsy, diabetes mellitus (with excretion of excess of fluid).

Investigations
Physical examination of abdomen and external genitalia.
Examination of urine for sugar, protein, micro-organisms, cells.
Occasionally X-ray examination of urinary tract, cystoscopy.

Treatment
1. Drug treatment. Antidepressants have been found to be effective in many cases. The drug of choice is imipramine in doses of 25 mg at night, increasing if necessary to 50 mg. The mode of action is not known. Treatment should be continued for several months. The dose can be cautiously reduced when the child has been continuously dry for a month. Relapse can occur. Other drugs used are amitryptiline and nortryptiline.

2. Conditioning with a pad-and-buzzer apparatus. In this apparatus a pad beneath the sheet on the child's bed is connected in an electrical circuit in such a way that as soon as the pad is wetted a bell is rung and the child wakes up. The child, being awoken every time he starts to wet the bed, develops in time a conditioned reflex against bed-wetting. There should be no restriction on the child's fluid intake, and he should not be lifted to be potted as this prevents the development of the reflex.

SOILING

Soiling (encopresis) is the passing of faeces into the clothes. A normal child is usually 'clean' by 3 years. Soiling after 4 is abnormal.

Causes

> mental handicap,
> inadequate and faulty training,

disturbed mother/child relationship,
regression during stressful period,
physical disease: constipation, anal fissure, Hirschprung's
disease.

Clinical picture
Boys are more commonly affected than girls. The soiling is usually by day, but it can occur at night.

Apart from the cases due to mental handicap, cases fall mainly into three groups.

1.   A social group with dull, inadequate or abnormal parents who have not trained their children properly. They come from a low socioeconomic group with a history of poverty, debt, bad housing, crime and unemployment.

2.   An aggressive soiling group, in which there is an obsessional, bowel-conscious mother who tries to train her child too early and too severely, and is obsessionally clean and tidy in other ways. The child can be well dressed and bright, and reacts to her mother with aggressive soiling, constipation and retention of faeces with over-flow.

3.   A regressive group in which the child responds by soiling when faced with a stress-producing situation. Other ways in which the child can respond are by bed-wetting and stammering.

Treatment
1.   Consistent and adequate training of the untrained.

2.   Psychotherapy of child and mother when the condition is due to an obsessional mother. Treatment of constipation by laxatives, enemas and suppositories is sometimes necessary, and the child may have to be admitted into hospital.

3.   Removal of stress-provoking factors and psychotherapy.

PICA

Pica is the eating by a child of stuff other than food. Toddlers normally try to eat things, but they stop if they are discouraged by their parents. Pica can be due to lack of training, mental handicap, autism, and severe conduct disorders. Paint, paper and dirt are commonly eaten; and a child can develop lead poisoning if he eats lead-containing paint.

Treatment is by treating the basic disorder in child and family.

BREATH-HOLDING

Breath-holding is a condition in which a child holds his breath until he goes blue in the face and falls unconscious. It usually starts before 2 years and stops at 5–6.

Breath-holding is precipitated by an attack of anger and crying. The child suddenly takes a deep breath and then stops breathing, becomes cyanosed and rigid, loses consciousness for a few moments, goes pale, relaxes and breathes again. Prolonged anoxia can cause a fit, but the incidence of epilepsy is no higher than in other children and the phenomenon is not thought to be an epileptic one. The child may be a tense, rigid one, and the parents may be overprotective. Occasionally the condition follows whooping cough. The only risk is of brain damage from prolonged anoxia.

Tics

Tics (habit spasms) are involuntary movements of groups of muscles. They are irregular and spasmodic, vary in degree of severity, and can recur hundreds of times a day. The face is usually affected, with eye-blinking as a common feature. Other parts of the body can be affected. The tics usually begin at about the age of 7, and more boys are affected than girls. Affected children may also show soiling, speech disorders and obsessional features.

The *cause* is unknown. Tics have been attributed to stress, developmental abnormalities and brain injury.

Treatment is by (a) removal of stress-provoking factors, (b) drugs, especially haloperidol and chlordiazepoxide, (c) psychotherapy, and (d) behaviour therapy.

Clumsy children

Some children are handicapped by extreme clumsiness. They have difficulty in performing movements, such as those involved in dressing, washing, walking, playing games, painting, handicrafts. Some have defective articulation. The handicap is likely to produce emotional difficulties, especially if the child is punished or ridiculed for his clumsiness. There is no clinical evidence of disease of the nervous and muscular systems. The condition appears to be a congenital disability to coordinate voluntary movements.

There is no specific treatment for the condition. It should be explained to the child, parents and teacher, and the child should be excused games and other physical activities which he cannot perform.

Stammering

Stammering (stuttering) can occur as a temporary condition due to anxiety, especially at 2–5 years when the child's ideas may outgrow his ability to express them in words. But stammering can be prolonged, severe, and persist in some degree into adult life. Some children talk with a stammer but sing without it; some stammer at school but not at home.

Precise causes are unknown. It is attributed to faulty parent/child relationships, anxiety, and brain damage involving the speech area. Without specific treatment stammering tends to disappear as the child grows older.

Treatment is unsatisfactory. It is by psychotherapy, removal from stress-provoking factors, and speech therapy.

Sleep-walking

Sleep-walking can be an expression of anxiety, be precipitated by nightmares or night terrors, or occur spontaneously. The child gets up and goes for a walk round the house or into the street. Sometimes he just stands by the bed or dresses himself. He may have a dim awareness of what is happening. He may put himself to bed without waking up. It is rare for a child to hurt himself while sleep-walking.

Nightmares and night terrors

Nightmares are unpleasant or frightening dreams. If the child is woken up, he behaves normally.

Night terrors occur commonly in young children. The child wakes up very frightened, does not reply to questions, does not appear to see things, talks as if other people were there, and is difficult to comfort. Eventually he goes to sleep and on awakening has no recollection of the incident.

Phobias

Phobias are exaggerated fears. It is normal for children to be afraid of some things—of the dark, of animals, of heights, etc; and fears should be considered abnormal only if they are severe, prolonged or multiple. A phobia may follow an actual fright, as a bitten child may be afraid of all dogs. A phobia can be the result of an emotional problem of which the child is unconscious, or of a fear that he will be punished for having feelings of hatred for a parent whom he usually loves.

School phobia (school refusal) is a phobia of going to school—or of leaving home. It is different from truancy, which is a wilful refusal to attend school.

Commonly at the time of going to school the child complains of abdominal pain, feeling sick or having diarrhoea. He becomes distressed if forced to go to school and can run away. He feels safe only at home. He is made worse by being forced to go to school, by bullies at school, a new or unsympathetic teacher. There may have been faulty parental attitudes.

Treatment is by home teaching and by psychotherapy of child and parents.

Elective mutism

In this condition a child will not speak away from home or in front of strangers. At home he talks freely. In the preschool period the child is usually regarded as shy. At school he will not speak to his teacher or other children, and he may not engage in games and other activities. He may show anxiety or appear in other respects normal.

Treatment is usually by some kind of psychotherapy, but is not very successful. Stress-provoking factors should, if present and possible, be removed.

Neuroses

ANXIETY STATES

Anxiety states in children differ from anxiety states in adults. The anxious child is commonly overactive and restless, and cannot sit still. He cannot give his attention to anything for long, and his school work suffers from this and because anxiety reduces learning ability. He can become tense and may bite his nails. He may be especially afraid of the dark, of being alone, of failing examinations. Sleep is often disturbed, and he may have nightmares or sleep-walk.

OBSESSIONAL-COMPULSIVE STATES

Some degree of obsessional thinking and compulsive behaviour can occur in healthy children, who can develop such compulsions as not stepping on the cracks in pavements, of jumping up steps in a particular order, of touching things. Such compulsions should not be considered abnormal unless they last a long time, seriously interfere with the child's normal activities, or start to appear in older children. Obsessional thoughts are that he has done wrong, is committing a sin, or should abuse his parents. The condition is particularly liable to occur in a child with obsessional-compulsive parents who has been trained to be always polite, clean and well behaved, to be always neatly dressed and immaculate. The child may develop soiling (encoporesis) as a reaction.

HYSTERIA

Hysteria is not very common in children. It can appear as paralysis, functional aphonia, amnesia, attacks of vomiting, diarrhoea or constipation, attacks of coughing, hiccoughing, and yawning, and attacks of frequency of micturition or polyuria, fainting. Some of these can spread like an epidemic through a group of children. An affected child may show *la belle indifférence*.

Psychosomatic disorders

Some psychosomatic disorders can occur in childhood.

Asthma can be produced by both allergic and psychological factors. Moreover a child with asthma is liable to develop anxiety during an attack and to be afraid of other attacks coming on. His parents usually become anxious and overprotective. The child dreads having an attack alone and away from his mother; and a suggestion from his mother that she might go away for a short time can be sufficient to bring on an attack.

Eczema can be due to allergic and emotional factors acting together. Children who have eczema in infancy often develop asthma and hay fever in later childhood.

Ulcerative colitis occurs in children as well as in adults. It is characterized by recurrent attacks of diarrhoea with blood-stained stools, with loss of appetite and wasting. It is difficult to treat and can ultimately cause death.

The cause is uncertain. Psychological factors have been incriminated. The child's parents may have given too much attention to bowel habits and been in the habit of giving him unnecessary purgatives. The child may have developed food fads and become obstinate and difficult to manage.

Psychoses

Psychoses are uncommon in childhood. They may be:

> autism,
> manic-depressive attacks,
> disintegrative psychosis.

AUTISM

Autism (childhood psychosis) develops in early childhood. The cause is unknown. It is usually attributed to a biochemical error of the brain or to some other error of cerebral function. There is a genetic factor: there is a higher incidence in identical twins than in non-identical twins. An unusually high proportion of the parents of an autistic child have a high intelligence.

In some children it seems to have been present since birth and these children show signs of it in early life. In other children it develops at 1–2 years, and in some others later still.

CLINICAL FEATURES

1. Loss of normal affection or non-development of it.
2. A failure of communication. The child does not learn to speak or stops if he has started. He may invent and use words of his own. He may show echolalia.
3. He seems to 'look through' people as if they were not there.
4. He does not play like a normal child nor with other children. He engages in apparently meaningless activities, such as twiddling a shoe-lace or running a toy car up and down a table for hours.

5. He may have attacks of acute excitement, in which he can mutilate himself. He usually does not attack other people.

6. He may recover if symptoms are mild and of short duration and can be attributed to a definite psychological factor (which is rare). Severely affected children do not recover.

TREATMENT

There is no satisfactory or specific treatment. The following are used in combination:

> special remedial education,
> psychotherapy,
> behaviour modification,
> tranquillizers.

Admission to a hospital for the mentally handicapped may be necessary. Some autistic children go to special residential homes and schools.

MANIC-DEPRESSIVE PSYCHOSIS

A manic-depressive psychosis is uncommon in childhood. Manic behaviour and hyperactivity can occur as well as depression. Cases clear up spontaneously or respond to family, work, environmental changes and psychotherapy.

DISINTEGRATIVE PSYCHOSIS

Disintegrative psychosis appears to be due to organic brain damage, e.g. by measles encephalitis and possibly by whooping-cough vaccine. The child had developed normally until illness damaged the brain. Clinical features are loss of speech, moodiness, negativism and aggression, and sometimes a progressive intellectual decline. The prognosis is poor. There is no specific treatment.

Brain damage

The brain of a child can be damaged in several ways.

1. Injury: at birth,   by baby battering,
               by road accidents,   by other accidents.

2. Infection: meningitis,   encephalitis.
            brain abscess,
3. Anoxia: during birth,   overdosage by sedative
            carbon monoxide   drugs.
            poisoning,
4. Cerebral tumour and degenerative disease, e.g. Huntingdon's chorea.

In addition to the disintegrative psychosis described above, an affected child can, according to the size and site of the damage, develop intellectual arrest, fits, paralysis, and speech disorders. The parents' emotional reaction to the damage can produce an emotional reaction in the child.

Hyperkinetic syndrome

In this condition the child is hyperactive and restless. It can become apparent when the child begins to walk. The child is constantly on the move. He cannot stay in one place, he cannot concentrate, is abnormally distractible, and is often aggressive and disobedient.

It can occur in children who show no signs of of brain damage. Others show some evidence of brain damage, commonly a slight defect of motor coordination. It can be associated with epilepsy and with depression.

Treatment is by haloperidol, a tranquillizer with orphenadrine to prevent the development of a drug-produced parkinsonism. Family therapy and psychotherapy concentrating on the mother/child relationship can be helpful.

Principles of treatment

Treatment of the mentally ill or disturbed child is by:

    individual psychotherapy,
    behaviour therapy,
    psychotherapy for sick or emotionally disturbed parents,
    family group therapy, in which the family is taken as the unit
        of treatment,
    modification of the child's environment at home,
    drugs: tranquillizers,

antidepressants,
anticonvulsants,
day patient care,
inpatient care,
educational changes: remedial teaching,
                    transfer to a special day or residential
                    school for disturbed children,
fostering,
care in a family group home or children's home.

Chapter 18 · Principles of treatment

In previous chapters indications have been given of the treatment for certain diseases. In this chapter will be described treatments applicable to many kinds of illness.

A nurse may feel frightened and at sea when she first has to look after patients suffering from mental illness. She has to face people with disordered minds who make great demands upon the nurse's time, patience, composure and intelligence, who may not accept her advice, refuse treatment and ordinary care, argue, act in peculiar ways, and sometimes physically oppose her ministrations. To the nursing of these patients the nurse must bring calmness, patience, confidence, firmness and an appreciation that the patient's irritability, negativism and hostility are expressions of illness. She must be willing to listen to the patient, to give encouragement, reassurance and an explanation of what she is doing.

Although the nurse should become a friend of the patient, she should not allow herself to be involved personally in the patient's problems. There is a danger in becoming too close a friend, in becoming emotionally as well as professionally attached, and it is important that the nurse should have interests of her own outside the hospital.

In hospital a nurse is much longer in contact with the patient than is the doctor. Her reports on the patient are of great importance to the doctor in making the diagnosis, choosing appropriate treatment, and assessing the effects of treatment and the fitness of the patient to leave hospital.

Hospitals and hostels

Some patients are looked after at home—when facilities are good, relationships with relatives are helpful, the administration of any drug is satisfactory, and the illness is not too acute, severe and antisocial.

If the patient has to go into hospital, the choice will be between a psychiatric ward in a general hospital and a ward in a psychiatric hospital. There are limitations to the kind of patient a general hospital can take. They are usually prepared to take patients for short-term care (up to a few months), they may not be equipped to take the most acute of patients, they may take only those patients for whom the outlook is good. There are advantages in the general hospital: it is more likely to be near the patient's home, he may feel less shame in going into it, and his relatives are more likely to agree. The psychiatric hospital will be prepared to provide any necessary kind of treatment and care for any kind of mental illness, and is likely to have recreational, occupational and industrial facilities on a scale not possible in the general hospital.

A *Day Hospital* is a small hospital or house to which patients come for the day. They spend the night and weekends at home. In this way the patient is not separated from his family, and the family is spared the difficulties of looking after him by day. A *Night Hospital* is a hospital to which the patient returns in the evening and where he sleeps. By day he is out at work or with his family. A *Hostel* is similar to a night hospital. It provides a place for the patient to live when he is convalescent and fit to go out to work, when he is suffering from a relatively mild illness but is not fit to look after himself, and when he has no home or when facilities at home are inadequate or relatives hostile or inadequate.

Facilities in hospitals

Some mental illnesses last a long time. They may be measured in months or years, and some may persist for the rest of the patient's life.

During the acute stage of his illness a patient has usually to be nursed in bed. If he is very disturbed in behaviour, he will have to be nursed in a single room with the furniture reduced to a minimum. When the acute phase of his illness is over, he will be allowed up. There has to be adequate space for patients to be up in, sitting rooms and dining rooms. The hospital provides the facilities by which the patient can be trained and encouraged to return to ordinary life and his work, and facilities for the welfare of patients who are not likely to be discharged. These facilities are likely to include:

occupational therapy,   art therapy,
industrial department,   physiotherapy,

music therapy,   physical training.

Psychotherapy

Psychotherapy is the treatment of illness essentially by listening and talking—by allowing the patient to talk and by talking to him—and by allowing emotional discharges. In a way every doctor and nurse practises psychotherapy whenever he listens and talks to a patient, but the term is used to describe more formal treatment as given by a psychiatrist or psychologist and sometimes also by a nurse therapist.

The purpose of psychotherapy is the development or restoration of mental and emotional health. One method is by allowing the patient to talk freely and describe his problems and emotional reactions. The psychotherapist reassures the patient, encourages him, suggests new ways of approaching his problems and coping with them or solving them.

Group therapy is a form of psychotherapy in which several patients are treated together, their problems and the ways in which they have failed or succeeded in solving them being openly discussed. Members of the group are encouraged to talk freely about their problems, emotional reactions are shared, and new methods of treatment discussed.

Psychodrama is an extension of group therapy. In it a group of patients act out a problem. The patient commonly acts his own life, with the other patients playing the roles of members of his family, his friends, his employer. No script is written, and the patient-actors develop the theme as they go along.

Abreaction is a method of liberating a patient's emotions and getting him to talk freely and without restraint by administering to him a drug likely to reduce his inhibitions, e.g. carbon dioxide, ether, or an intravenous barbiturate. It is hoped that in this way inhibitions are abolished and the patient's underlying thoughts and emotions given a chance of expression. Abreactive techniques can be used for both diagnostic and therapeutic purposes.

Behaviour therapy is a method of training patients in socially acceptable behaviour and abolishing socially unacceptable behaviour, and in the treatment of phobias and drug addiction. The principles involved are the rewarding of good behaviour and the punishing or not rewarding of bad behaviour. To change any behaviour, the behaviour must be followed by a reinforcer, which to have the maximum effect must immediately follow the behaviour. The reinforcement must be given every time the behaviour occurs, and all staff concerned with the treatment of the patient must be trained in the techniques.

Hypnosis is a form of suggestion used in the treatment of hysteria and some other conditions. The patient is put into a hypnotic state by the doctor who suggests that he should pass into a deep sleep while still being aware of the doctor's voice and obeying his instructions. Some patients (especially hysterics and physically exhausted people) are more suggestible than others. Under hypnosis the patient is instructed to use a hysterically paralysed limb or to regain a hysterically lost voice, and he may be given post-hypnotic suggestions as to what he should do on awakening.

Analysis is a more formal method of psychotherapy, and its exponents consider it the only method. Techniques vary according to whether the analyst is a follower of Freud or Jung. The patient usually attends once or twice a week, and treatment may have to continue for years. He lies on a couch and talks to the analyst. In the course of talking in the method of 'free association' (in which the patient talks about whatever comes into his head, regardless of any apparent connection it may or may not have with the troubles he is being treated for), he comes to talk about matters he has forgotten, especially those affecting his childhood, his relations with his parents, his early emotional problems. In this way he exposes much forgotten material from his unconscious life and he may liberate emotional forces, turning them upon his analyst, who may for a time stand as a representative of a parent. According to his school of psychotherapy, the analyst either listens passively and interprets material or takes a more suggestive role, indicating to the patient what he thinks he should do about it.

The care of the acute patient

Whatever the cause of the illness, the acute mental patient presents serious nursing problems.

On admission the patient may be excited, unreasonable, confused, destructive, assaultive or suicidal. Treatment in a single room is essential at first. For very acute patients the bedstead may have to be removed and the patient nursed on a mattress and bedclothes on the floor. It is usually necessary to remove spectacles and dentures. Daily bathing and attention to mouth, teeth, nails, hair and skin are necessary.

If a patient is regarded as dangerous, a nurse should not go in alone to him. She may be attacked if she does. She should wait until assistance is available; a patient may accept treatment without much resistance if he finds three or four nurses around him. If a nurse happens to be alone with a patient who becomes threatening or dangerous, she should not turn her back on him and should try to see that he does not get between her and the door.

If a patient is regarded as suicidal, special precautions have to be taken. He should be examined to ensure that he has not in his possession or in his clothes anything with which he might commit suicide. He should not be allowed out of the nurse's sight; he should not be left alone in a ward nor allowed to go alone to the toilet or bathroom. He should not be allowed to shave himself, should not be allowed near surgical instruments or drugs, nor should he be left alone in a kitchen or garden. One of the biggest problems in the care of a patient is the assessment of whether he has ceased to be suicidal, and a time may come when the doctor decides that a risk has to be taken.

The patient may not drink or eat enough. He may be too confused or excited to take food, depressed and unwilling to live, or deluded that the food is poisoned. The nurse must try by persuasion and patience to get him to take enough, and he may have to be spoon-fed. A few applications of ECT may start him eating again.

An acutely ill patient can become constipated. Less mess is caused and no dehydration if he is given an enema and not a purgative. Faecal impaction can occur, especially in senile patients. An olive oil enema is given, or the impacted faeces removed manually. If urinary retention occurs, an attempt is made to have the patient empty his bladder while having a hot bath; if this fails, he has to be catheterized.

The acutely ill patient requires rest, sleep, and relief from any depressive ideas he may have. The available drugs are:

sedatives and hypnotics,
tranquillizers,
antidepressants.

Hypnotics and sedatives

These drugs are given to produce sleep and rest. They are classified in two groups: the non-barbiturates and the barbiturates.

(a) NON-BARBITURATES

Chloral hydrate: dose 300 mg—2 g; safe; few side effects; suitable for the frail and elderly.
Dichloralphenazone (Welldorm): dose 600 mg–1.8 g.
Triclofos sodium (Tricloryl): dose 500 mg–2.0 g.
Glutethimide (Doriden): dose 250–500 mg; can cause nausea and purpura.
Nitrazepam (Mogadon): dose 5–10 mg, 2.5–5 mg for elderly patients.
Paraldehyde: dose 2–10 ml by mouth or intramuscular injection; safe, rapidly acting; very unpleasant taste and smell; dissolves plastic syringes; can cause abscess at site of injection.

(b) BARBITURATES

Although many people take them without ill effects, barbiturates can become drugs of addiction, cause death by depressing the circulatory and respiratory centres in the brain, have serious interactions with other drugs by interfering with liver function, and by accumulation in the body produce a chronic cerebral condition with drowsiness, disorientation, confusion, ataxia and slurred speech.
Amylobarbitone sodium (Sodium Amytal): dose 100–200 mg.
Butobarbitone (Soneryl): dose 100–200 mg.
Pentobarbitone sodium (Nembutal): dose 100–200 mg.

Tranquillizers

Tranquillizers are used to control excitement, overactivity, and irritability, and to promote sleep, in patients suffering from anxiety states, mania, schizophrenia, dementia, etc. There are many such drugs on the market.
Chlorpromazine (Largactil): dose 15–50 mg daily, increasing up to 1000 mg daily in divided doses for severe illness; toxic effects

include drowsiness, hypotension, parkinsonism, jaundice, skin rashes, skin discoloration.

Trifluoperazine (Stelazine): dose 15–30 mg daily by mouth, 1–3 mg by intramuscular injection.

Haloperidol: dose can be low-starting 750 μg daily, increasing, or high-starting 15 mg daily, reducing; can produce parkinsonism.

Thioridazine (Melleril): dose 30–600 mg daily in divided doses; can produce drowsiness, dizziness, dryness of mouth.

Drug-induced parkinsonism can be prevented and treated by anti-parkinsonism drugs, such as benxhexol (Artane), benztropin (Cogentin), and procyclidine (Kemadrin).

Antidepressants

Antidepressants are used in the treatment of depression of all kinds. There are many on the market.

Amitriptyline (Lentizol, Saroten, Tryptizol: dose up to 150 mg daily in divided doses, for patients over 60 up to 90 mg daily; can produce drowsiness, constipation, headache, dizziness, shaking of limbs, obesity, parkinsonism, paralytic ileus, etc.

Imipramine (Berkomine, Norpramine, Tofranil): dose 75–150 mg daily in divided doses, for patients over 60 up to 90 mg daily; toxic effects similar to those of amitriptyline.

Nortriptyline (Allegron, Aventyl): dose 20–100 mg daily in divided doses, toxic effects similar to those of amitriptyline.

Chlordiazepoxide (Librium, Tropium): dose 30–100 mg daily in divided doses; also used to prevent recurrent attacks of depression and mania.

Drugs of the MAOI group (monoamine oxidase inhibitors) are used as antidepressants. They can interact seriously with other drugs and with certain foods—cheese, yoghurt, broad beans, Bovril, Marmite—and with alcohol. They include:

phenelzine (Nardil): dose 15–75 mg daily in divided doses;

tranylcypromine (Parnate): dose 20–30 mg daily in divided doses;

isocarboxazid (Marplan): dose up to 30 mg daily in divided doses.

Electroconvulsive treatment

Electroconvulsive treatment (ECT) is a method of treatment of mental illness by the passing of an electrical current through the prefrontal lobes of the brain. As originally given, ECT produced a major epileptic fit, with all the complications of a major fit. ECT is now usually given under an anaesthetic and with an intravenous muscle relaxant drug, so that only very slight twitching at the most is produced.

The patient should not have had any food for several hours. He is given atropine 1.2 mg 30 minutes before treatment to reduce salivation. His bladder should be empty and his clothing loose. Dentures, spectacles and metal hair-grips are removed. The patient lies on a couch or firm bed. The anaesthetist administers the intravenous anaesthetic and muscle relaxant. The doctor then administers the electrical current from a machine designed for the purpose through electrodes soaked in saline and applied to the patient's temples. From 70 to 130 volts for 0.1–0.5 seconds are necessary. The patient may twitch a little round his mouth and eyes; to hold him is unnecessary. The anaesthetist will maintain the patient's blood oxygenated with an oxygen insufflator until the action of the muscle relaxant wears off and the patient starts to breathe again. He is allowed to rest until he recovers completely. He may complain of malaise, headache, nausea or giddiness.

Unilateral ECT is thought to cause less confusion and memory loss. It is applied to the non-dominant cerebral hemisphere, but it is not easy to establish which this is. The two electrodes are applied to the same side of the head, one 4 cm above the midpoint between the external angle of the eye and the earhole and the other 9 cm away vertically above the earhole.

ECT is used in the treatment of:

> severe depression,
> acute excitement, manic or schizophrenic,
> catatonic stupor,
> confusional states.

Treatment is given daily or two or three times a week. The number given varies with the patient's response, but a course is not usually more than eight. It can be given to an outpatient, but a relative or friend should accompany the patient home.

Contraindication: a recent coronary thrombosis.

Complications:

> headache, malaise, nausea, giddiness,
> prolonged muscular paralysis,
> laryngeal spasm,

loss of memory, inability to concentrate,
conversion of depression into mania.

Modified insulin treatment

Modified insulin treatment is so-called because it is a modification of the deep insulin treatment once used for schizophrenia. It is used in the treatment of anxiety states and anorexia nervosa.

Treatment is given daily for 5–6 days a week for a month or until the patient has regained her normal weight. Each morning the patient is given fasting an intramuscular dose of insulin, beginning with 10 units and increasing to 100 units if necessary. The aim is to produce a mild hypoglycaemia, the symptoms of which are hunger, sweating and drowsiness. The patient remains in bed in a darkened room. After 2–3 hours the hypoglycaemia is stopped by giving the patient a sugared drink and a large breakfast with added carbohydrate. She should be kept under observation for the rest of the day.

Complications:

hypoglycaemia later in the day,
coma,
fit.

Prefrontal leucotomy

In the operation of prefrontal leucotomy (USA: lobotomy) some of the nerve fibres connecting the prefrontal lobes of the brain with the thalamus on either side are divided. There are several types of operation, the aim of which is to produce the best result with the minimum of complications. It is used for:

severe chronic stress, anxiety and agitation, whatever the cause,
anorexia nervosa,
spasmodic torticollis,

when other methods of treatment have failed, when there is little likelihood of the patient recovering spontaneously, when his life has been made intolerable, or when death seems otherwise likely.

The mortality from the operation is about 3 per cent, from cerebral haemorrhage. Complications are:

apathy,
disregard of social conventions,
fits,
urinary incontinence.

The care of the chronic patient

A number of patients develop chronic illnesses and have to be looked after in one way or another for life. If symptoms are mild, relatives are available, cooperative and understanding, and the patient's behaviour socially acceptable, he may be looked after at home and attend a day hospital or facilities provided by the local authority. But many long-term patients have to live in hospital.

A nurse should ensure that her patients are as far as possible clean and tidy, and she should train them from the first in good habits. She should make sure that they wash and bath adequately, brush their hair, and keep their clothes clean and tidy. Male patients should be shaved daily unless they wear a beard. Eccentricities of dress and personal adornment should be checked.

Patients should be encouraged to keep their ward or villa clean and tidy—it is their home—and to make beds, lay tables and wash up. Each patient should have a particular task assigned to him, and care has to be taken that one patient does not encroach on another's territory. Patients who quarrel or fight have to be kept apart from each other.

So far as is possible the patient should be engaged in some form of activity and occupation; he should be given enough to help and stimulate him, but he can suffer from having too much as well as from having too little. Psychiatric hospitals provide facilities for industrial work of various kinds, occupational or recreational therapy, art therapy, music therapy, and gardening. The patients may run their own Social Club, and there may be a special club for the elderly.

Legal requirements in England and Wales

Most patients are admitted into hospital as informal patients. All they have to do is to express a wish to go in, or if taken to the hospital agree to go in. As informal patients they have the same rights as other people, can refuse treatment, can discharge themselves on their own account or be discharged by the hospital.

As it is necessary to admit some patients compulsorily and against their will, their legal status is controlled by law. The Mental Health Act, 1959, defines mental disorders and states how patients may be admitted, kept there, and be discharged. It makes the following definitions:

(a) *Mental disorder* is defined as 'mental illness, arrested or incomplete development of mind, psychopathic disorder, and any other disorder or disability of mind'.

(b) *Severe subnormality* is defined as 'a state of arrested or incomplete development of mind which includes subnormality of intelligence and is of such a nature or degree that the patient is incapable of living an independent life or of guarding himself against serious exploitation, or will be so when of an age to do so'.

(c) *Subnormality* is defined as 'a state of arrested or incomplete development of mind (not amounting to severe subnormality) which includes subnormality of intelligence and is of a nature or degree which requires or is susceptible to medical treatment or other special care or training of the patient'.

(d) *Psychopathic disorder* is defined as 'persistent disorder or disability of mind (whether or not including subnormality of intelligence) which results in abnormally aggressive or seriously irresponsible conduct on the part of the patient, and requires or is susceptible to medical treatment'.

The Act makes no attempt to define 'mental illness', has introduced the clumsy and unfortunately chosen terms of 'subnormality' and 'severe subnormality' to describe what is more acceptably known as mental handicap or retardation, and makes a particularly bad description of psychopathic disorder for many psychopaths are unaffected by any form of medical treatment. What rights over treatment and care the compulsorily detained patient has are not clear.

The Act was, however, reviewed in 1978, and a Government White Paper published setting out proposals for change, based on the need 'to strengthen the rights and safeguard the liberties of the mentally disordered whilst retaining a proper regard for the rights and safety of the general public and of staff'.

The law relating to the compulsory admission of patients is complex. In general, a patient can be admitted compulsorily into any hospital or mental nursing home willing to take him on an application made in writing by the nearest relative or by an appropriate officer of the local authority in whose area he is living, with the written recommendations of two doctors, one of whom has special knowledge of psychiatry and has been approved by a local authority.

The patient may be admitted either for *observation* for 28 days or for *treatment*, in which case the compulsion can last for up to one year and if necessary can then be renewed. If he has been admitted for *observation*, he can within the 28 days' detention become an informal patient or a further application for his detention for *treatment* can be made so that he may be detained longer. For urgent cases one medical recommendation, in addition to the application, is sufficient for the patient's admission, but a second medical recommendation must be obtained within 72 hours.

The patient may be discharged by the consultant psychiatrist (who is called the responsible medical officer) in charge of him, by his nearest relative, or by the governing body of the hospital. There are special provisions by which the discharge of a dangerous patient can be prevented. Certain courts can commit to hospital a person who has while suffering from mental disorder committed an offence for which imprisonment can be a punishment; and there are special restrictions on the discharge of a patient who has committed a very serious offence who can be discharged only with the approval of the Home Secretary. At certain specified times a compulsorily detained patient or his nearest relative can appeal to a Mental Health Review Tribunal for his discharge.

Index

abreaction 121
absences 65–6
activity, in mental illness 6–7
acute patient, care of 122
affect, incongruity of 7
affective psychoses 25–31
agoraphobia 13
akinetic epilepsy 67
alcohol 44
  clinical features of dependence
    on 45–6
alcoholic hallucinosis 47, 49
alcoholics, personality of 45
alcoholism 44–9
  chronic 47–8
  diseases of 46–8
  incidence of 44–5
  and mental handicap 48, 105
  prevention of 48
  treatment of 48–9
Alzheimer's disease 74–5
amnesia 9
  hysterical 16
  post-traumatic 55
  retrograde 54–5
amphetamine addiction 51–2
anaesthesia, hysterical 15
analysis 122
anorexia nervosa 20–1
anoxia 85, 97
antidepressive drugs 28–9, 125
anxiety states 11–13
  in childhood 113–14
aphonia, hysterical 15
Argyll-Robertson pupil 58
arsonist 42
arteriosclerotic dementia 79–80
asthma 22–3, 114
autism 115–16
automatic obedience 6

barbiturates 124
  addiction to 50–1
bed-wetting 108–9
behaviour, antisocial 9–10
  criminal 9–10
  in schizophrenia 35

behaviour therapy 121–2
belle indifférence, la 14, 114
blindness, hysterical 15
blocking, of talk 8
brain damage, in childhood 116–17
  and mental handicap 105
  psychiatric results of 54–7
breath-holding 111
bromide poisoning 92

cannabis addiction 52–3
cerebral palsy 99–100
cerebral tumour 88–9
childbearing, mental disorders of 93
childhood, brain damage in 116–17
  conduct disorders in 108–13
  neuroses in 113–14
  psychiatry of 3, 117–18
  psychosis in 115–17
  psychosomatic disorders in
    114–15
  treatment in 117–18
chronic patient, care of 128
circumstantiality 8
clang association 7
claustrophobia 13
clumsy children 111–12
cocaine addiction 52
coma 9
concussion 54–5
conduct, in mental illness 5
conduct disorders in childhood
  108–13
confabulation 9
confusion 9
confusional state, in arteriosclerotic
  dementia 79
  in old age 81
  in senile dementia 78
consciousness, disturbances of 9
conversion reactions 14–15
coronary thrombosis 23
corpus callosum, division of 71
cretinism 103
Cushing's syndrome 87–8
cytomegalovirus infection 101–2